AF713369

BRAIN COMPUTER INTERFACE

BRAIN COMPUTER INTERFACE

EEG Signal Processing

Narayan Panigrahi and Saraju P. Mohanty

CRC Press
Taylor & Francis Group
Boca Raton London New York

CRC Press is an imprint of the
Taylor & Francis Group, an **informa** business

MATLAB® is a trademark of The MathWorks, Inc. and is used with permission. The MathWorks does not warrant the accuracy of the text or exercises in this book. This book's use or discussion of MATLAB® software or related products does not constitute endorsement or sponsorship by The MathWorks of a particular pedagogical approach or particular use of the MATLAB® software

First edition published 2023
by CRC Press
6000 Broken Sound Parkway NW, Suite 300, Boca Raton, FL 33487-2742

and by CRC Press
2 Park Square, Milton Park, Abingdon, Oxon, OX14 4RN

© 2023 Narayan Panigrahi and Saraju P. Mohanty

CRC Press is an imprint of Taylor & Francis Group, LLC

Reasonable efforts have been made to publish reliable data and information, but the author and publisher cannot assume responsibility for the validity of all materials or the consequences of their use. The authors and publishers have attempted to trace the copyright holders of all material reproduced in this publication and apologize to copyright holders if permission to publish in this form has not been obtained. If any copyright material has not been acknowledged please write and let us know so we may rectify in any future reprint.

Except as permitted under U.S. Copyright Law, no part of this book may be reprinted, reproduced, transmitted, or utilized in any form by any electronic, mechanical, or other means, now known or hereafter invented, including photocopying, microfilming, and recording, or in any information storage or retrieval system, without written permission from the publishers.

For permission to photocopy or use material electronically from this work, access www.copyright.com or contact the Copyright Clearance Center, Inc. (CCC), 222 Rosewood Drive, Danvers, MA 01923, 978-750-8400. For works that are not available on CCC please contact mpkbookspermissions@tandf.co.uk

Trademark notice: Product or corporate names may be trademarks or registered trademarks and are used only for identification and explanation without intent to infringe.

Library of Congress Cataloging-in-Publication Data
A catalog record has been requested for this book

ISBN: 978-1-032-14841-0 (hbk)
ISBN: 978-1-032-14842-7 (pbk)
ISBN: 978-1-003-24138-6 (ebk)

DOI: 10.1201/9781003241386

Typeset in Times
by MPS Limited, Dehradun

Contents

Preface

Brain computer interface, popularly known as BCI, is an emerging field of research, finding its use in many societal and medical applications. BCI comprises of four distinct steps: (1) neuro-imaging for acquisition of the digital data from the brain, (2) processing of the neuro-image data for isolating various characteristic features of the brain, (3) classification and mapping of the features to understand the intended motif and actions, and (4) interfacing the action to the device or computer to perform the intended actions. There is more than one method to perform each of these steps. Also, there is directed research to innovate and optimize these methods to make these steps efficient and autonomous in achieving BCI.

In this book, we choose electroencephalography (EEG) as the neuro-imaging technique for performing the data acquisition for BCI. In the rest of the steps the algorithms, computing techniques, visualization, and interpretation of features extracted from EEG were discussed. Therefore, this is the name of the book *Brain Computer Interface: EEG Signal Processing*. EEG has many spatio-temporal variations and has different ways to acquire an EEG signal. Matching computing techniques and interpretation methods are being researched upon so as to make use of these spatio-temporal variations. The features extracted from EEG are exploited in actuation of devices and computers so as to realize the BCI. Another aspect of neuro-imaging signature of the brain is observed to be fairly similar when a subject performs a similar task but differs in the level for different activities.

We believe that EEG signals, if processed using the right methodology, will help in determining the cognitive behavior of a subject. One aspect of the cognitive behavior is intelligence. As mentioned earlier, the EEG signals are the signature of the brain activity of different regions of the subject.

This book gives a basic introduction to various neuro-imaging techniques, with a special emphasis to EEG and its advantages. Further, the basic classification criteria for different components present in EEG are discussed. It gives varying perspectives as how to understand the scope of processing the EEG signal and its association with popular applications.

The signal processing methods that are useful in processing and identifying EEG artifacts to detect the blinks, saccadic movements, and fixes in the EEG data are discussed. Classification of EEG signals for detection of target or non-target objects was determined based on the presence of P300 signal while acquiring the EEG while the subject is exposed to a corresponding scenario or probe. The saccadic movement fixes and the blinks determine the focus and way in which the subject scan through the scene or the scenario placed in his/her view.

In a recent development, EEG has proven to bring out new insights related to the activity of the brain in a non-invasive manner. It is used in different applications to measure the intended effect of any activity that the subject performs or any stimuli that is given to the subject. With the help of artificial intelligence, analysis of EEG has reached a new level as it allows us to perform intractable operations that were otherwise not possible using classical techniques. In the area of neuro-marketing, it has given a deeper insight so as to how consumers react to certain products. In the medical field, prior prediction of seizures in epileptic patients is progressing rapidly. In military applications, the EEG is used to measure the responsiveness of the candidate under examinations. The most popular area of application of EEG is brain controlled interface (BCI), where devices are being controlled with the help of the brain signals.

In this book, we have discussed selected signal processing methods to extract the blink, saccade, and fix artifacts from the EEG signal obtained from different subjects.

Further, this book discusses and proposes a design to build a low-cost yet robust EEG acquisition system that has all the elements from acquisition of the EEG to its processing and visualization. The students will benefit immensely to build and experiment with such a system ab-initio. Some of the interesting applications derived by processing the EEG and electrooculography (EOG) signal were discussed to make the reading more interesting.

Processing and analyzing the P300 signal using odd-ball experiments makes this book more interesting. The basis of EEG being the key elements of BCI (brain computer interface) is discussed. Further, how to detect and classify abnormal EEG signals such as epileptic seizure is discussed for students perusing research in the field of IoMT (Internet of medical things).

For a quick benefit to the students and research community, we append some of the MATLAB® codes illustrating how to process, analyze, and visualize the EEG signal and the artifacts present in EEG. A quick run of these MATLAB® codes will help the reader to consolidate some of the key concepts explained in this book.

Narayan Panigrahi and Saraju P. Mohanty

MATLAB® is a trademark of The MathWorks, Inc. and is used with permission. The MathWorks does not warrant the accuracy of the text or exercises in this book. This book's use or discussion of MATLAB® software or related products does not constitute endorsement or sponsorship by The MathWorks of a particular pedagogical approach or particular use of the MATLAB® software.

Authors

Narayan Panigrahi received his MSc (computer science) from the J.K. Institute of Applied Physics & Technology, University of Allahabad; M.Tech (computer science and data processing), IIT, Kharagpur; and PhD from IIT, Bombay in the years 1990, 1999, and 2012, respectively. He is the best graduate of Berhampur University, Odisha, in the year 1987. He started as a research scientist at the Institute for System Studies and Analysis (ISSA), New Delhi, in the year 1991. He initiated research and development of modeling and visualization of topography, bathymetry, and space. Currently, he is serving as a scientist at the Center for Artificial Intelligence and Robotics (CAIR), a DRDO Laboratory in Bangalore, India. He leads a team of scientists to design and develop a geographical information system comprising of topography, bathymetry, and space navigation. He has researched the algorithmic aspect of remote sensing, spatio-temporal science, and GIS. He has initiated communication of science through authoring various books in different languages. He has authored *Geographic Information Science (GISc)* (CRC Press, 2009) and *Computating in Geographic Information Systems* (CRC Press, 2014), which are being taught in different academic circles. He has been awarded the "National Award for Geospatial Excellence 2019" from the ISRS (Indian Society for Remote Sensing), Agni Award for Excellence in Self Reliance -2019, DRDO Performance Excellence Award 2012, and Laboratory Technology Award for 2010, 2014, 2017, and 2019, respectively. He has uthored seven books, 72 international research papers, and six patents. Two of his research papers were awarded best research award by INRIA, France and IEEE, Computer Society. He has examined 5 PhD thesis, guided more than 40 graduate and undergraduate engineering students. He is a plenary and invited speaker in many international conferences and has chaired technical sessions.

Saraju P. Mohanty received B. Tech. (Honors) in electrical engineering from the Orissa University of Agriculture and Technology, Bhubaneswar, in 1995; master's degree in systems science and automation from the Indian Institute of Science, Bengaluru, in 1999; and PhD degree in computer science and engineering from the University of South Florida, Tampa, in 2003. He is a professor with the University of North Texas. His research is in smart electronic systems, which has been funded by National Science Foundations (NSF), Semiconductor Research Corporation (SRC), U.S. Air Force, IUSSTF, and Mission Innovation. He has authored 350 research articles, four books, and invented four granted and one pending patents. His Google Scholar h-index is 38 and i10-index is 147, with 6,600 citations. He is regarded as a visionary researcher on smart cities technology in which his research deals with security and energy awareness and AI/ML-integrated smart components. He introduced the secure digital camera (SDC) in 2004 with built-in security features designed using hardware-assisted security (HAS) or security by design (SbD) principle.

He is widely credited as the designer for the first digital watermarking chip in 2004 and first for the low-power digital watermarking chip in 2006. He is a recipient of 12 best paper awards, Fulbright Specialist Award in 2020, IEEE Consumer Technology Society Outstanding Service Award in 2020, the IEEE-CS-TCVLSI Distinguished Leadership Award in 2018, and the PROSE Award for Best Textbook in Physical Sciences and Mathematics category in 2016. He has delivered ten keynotes and served on nine panels at various international conferences. He has been serving on the editorial board of several peer-reviewed international journals. He has mentored two post-doctoral researchers, and supervised 12 PhD dissertations, 26 M.S. theses, and ten undergraduate projects.

1 Introduction

OVERVIEW

Electroencephalography, or EEG, is one of the best and oldest non-invasive neuro-scanning methods. The EEG is also the most preferred one of the foremost choices for doctors and surgeons for diagnosis of neuro- or brain-related ailments. With the advent of modern computing algorithms, the traditional EEG is under metamorphosis. Many novel systems are being devised using EEG and computing methods innovating different systems. Some of the prominent applications of EEG are brain computer interface (BCI), neuro-marketing, gaming, and pre-detection and diagnosis of seizures are widely used. This chapter introduces the EEG to the first-time reader of this book with a general definition of EEG. It analyzes the systemic and functional perspective of a human brain. Further, it gives a survey of prominent neuro-scanning systems comparing and contrasting these systems with EEG. The normal characteristic of the EEG signal acquired from the human brain is discussed and analyzed. Based on the signal characteristic, the physical interpretation of the state of the subject is classified. To motivate the first-time reader of this book, some popular medical and commercial applications are also discussed in this chapter. Some of the basic questions regarding EEG are answered in this introductory chapter, including "What is an EEG?" and "Why is an EEG performed?"

1.1 THE HUMAN BRAIN

Since this book deals with characterization of the human brain through the EEG signal acquired from the brain for the purpose of BCI (brain computer interface), therefore, it is pertinent to understand the anatomy, structure, and functioning of the human brain.

The brain is the vital organ that controls all functions of the body, it interprets information from the outside world, and embodies the essence of the mind and soul. Intelligence, creativity, emotion, and memory are a few of the many functions governed by the brain. Protected within the skull, the brain is composed of the cerebrum, cerebellum, and brain stem.

The brain receives information through our five senses: sight, smell, touch, taste, and hearing – often simultaneously. It collates and stores this information in our memory the messages in a way that has a lasting meaning for us. The brain controls our thoughts, memory, and speech; movement of the arms and legs; and the function of many organs within our body. It performs some directed or voluntary functions and some involuntary functions of the body.

DOI: 10.1201/9781003241386-1

The brain consists of trillions (*approx* $\sim 2^{18}$ *for a healthy adult*) of cells, half of which are neurons and the other half of which help and facilitate conducting the signal among neurons and the rest are controlling the activity of neurons. The neurons are densely interconnected via synapses, which act as gateways of inhibitory or excitatory activities of the brain.

1.2 ANATOMY OF HUMAN BRAIN

The human brain is one of the most complex and specialized parts of the human body. It has many parts and each of these parts is associated with different functions performed by human. Therefore, to characterize the brain and analyze its structural, functional, and control behavior, it is necessary to study its anatomy. An anatomically human brain is organized into four parts: (1) forebrain, (2) midbrain, (3) hindbrain, and (4) the skull, which is also known as the cranium or the brain box.

Systematically the brain can be categorized into three subparts. Each subpart has different sub-subparts and performs specific functions, as depicted in Figure 1.1. Further, the lateral view (Figure 1.2(a)) and the systemic view (Figure 1.2(b)) give an overview of the anatomy of the human brain.

The central nervous system (CNS) is composed of the brain and spinal cord. The peripheral nervous system (PNS) is composed of spinal nerves that branch from the spinal cord and cranial nerves that branch from the brain. The three main parts of the central nervous system are the (1) cerebrum, (2) cerebellum, and (3) brain stem.

1. **Cerebrum** is the largest part of the brain and is composed of right and left hemispheres. It performs all cognitive functions like interpreting touch, vision and hearing, as well as speech, reasoning, emotions, learning, and fine control of movement. Also it retains the experiences in the form of memory.

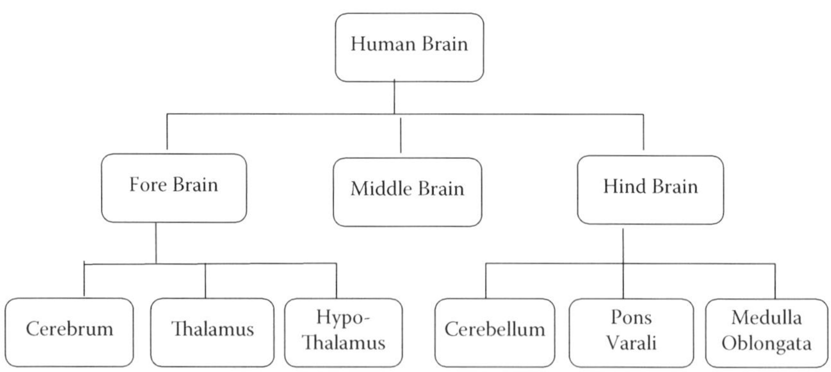

FIGURE 1.1 Hierarchical view of the functional parts and sub-parts of the brain.

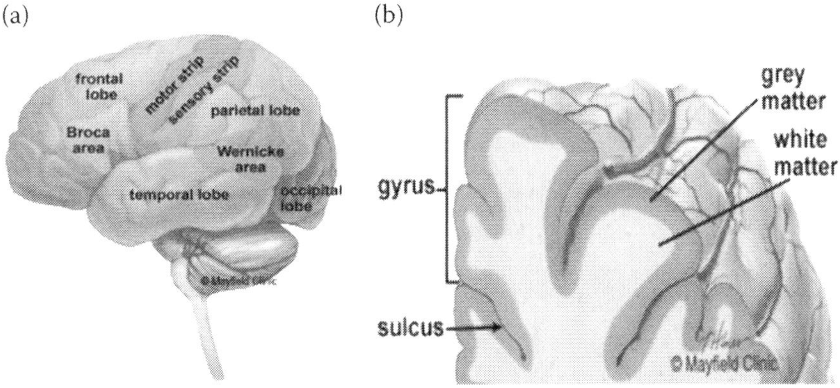

FIGURE 1.2 (a) The cerebrum is divided into four lobes: frontal, parietal, occipital, and temporal (b) The cortex contains neurons (grey matter), which are interconnected to other brain areas by axons (white matter). The cortex has a folded appearance. A fold is called a gyrus and the valley between is a sulcus.

2. **Cerebellum** is located under the cerebrum. Its function is to coordinate muscle movements, maintain posture, and balance (Apps & Garwicz 2005).
3. **Brain stem** acts as a relay center as well as the manager of the brain. It connects the cerebrum and cerebellum to the spinal cord. It performs many automatic functions such as breathing, heart rate, body temperature, wake and sleep cycles, digestion, sneezing, coughing, vomiting, and swallowing.

Further, the cerebrum is divided into two halves: the left cerebrum and right cerebrum are often loosely referred as the right brain and left brain or the right and left hemispheres (Figure 1.2(b)). They are joined by a bundle of fibers called the corpus callosum that transmits messages from one side to the other. Each hemisphere controls the opposite side of the body. If a stroke occurs on the right side of the brain, the left arm or leg may be weak or will be paralyzed.

Not all functions of the hemispheres are shared. In general, the left hemisphere controls speech, comprehension, arithmetic, and writing. The right hemisphere controls creativity, spatial ability, artistic, and musical skills. Generally, the left hemisphere is dominant in hand use and the right hemisphere controls use language in about 92% of people.

1.3 DIFFERENT BRAIN LOBES AND THEIR FUNCTIONS

Further the brain is subdivided into various clusters known as lobes housing various glands and ventricles. The cerebral hemispheres have distinct fissures, which divide the brain into lobes. Each hemisphere has four lobes: frontal, temporal, parietal, and occipital (Figure 1.2(a)). Each lobe may be further divided, into areas that serve very specific functions. It's important to understand that each lobe of the brain does not function alone. There are very complex relationships between the lobes of the brain and between the right and left hemispheres.

a. **Frontal Lobe**
   - Personality, behavior, emotions
   - Judgment, planning, problem solving
   - Speech: speaking and writing (Broca's area)
   - Body movement (motor strip)
   - Intelligence, concentration, self awareness
b. **Parietal Lobe**
   - Interprets language, words
   - Sense of touch, pain, temperature (sensory strip)
   - Interprets signals from vision, hearing, motor, sensory, and memory
   - Spatial and visual perception
c. **Occipital Lobe**
   - Interprets vision (color, light, movement)
d. **Temporal Lobe**
   - Understanding language (Wernicke's area)
   - Memory
   - Hearing
   - Sequencing and organization

Therefore, while designing an EEG acquisition system, it is important to provision a proportionate number of electrodes to probe each of the functional lobes of the brain and designate the signals acquired. The corresponding signals can be processed to diagnose the ailments and functioning of that part of the brain. Also, it helps in segregating different signal characteristics for different commands intended from the brain. Therefore, a study of the EEG signals as per different brain lobes helps in designing an efficient brain-computer interface.

1.4 FUNCTIONAL OVERVIEW OF BRAIN

1.4.1 Language and Memory Functions

How the special functions and involuntary and voluntary functions are governed by the brain are well researched. Language, memory, and speech are some of the special functions that are governed by different parts of the brain. If these areas malfunction, then they result in aberrations such as aphasia and other speech-related difficulties. The left hemisphere of the brain is responsible for language and speech and is called the "dominant" hemisphere. The right hemisphere plays a large part in interpreting visual information and spatial processing. In about one-third of people who are left-handed, speech function may be located on the right side of the brain. Left-handed people may need special testing to determine if their speech center is on the left or right side prior to any surgery in that area.

Aphasia is a disturbance of language affecting speech production, comprehension, reading or writing, due to brain injury – most commonly from stroke or trauma. The type of aphasia depends on the brain area damaged.

- **Broca's area:** lies in the left frontal lobe (Figure 1.2(a)). If this area is damaged, one may have difficulty moving the tongue or facial muscles to produce the sounds of speech. The person can still read and understand spoken language, but has difficulty in speaking and writing (i.e., forming letters and words, doesn't write within lines) – called Broca's aphasia.
- **Wernicke's area:** lies in the left temporal lobe (Figure 1.2(a)). Damage to this area causes Wernicke's aphasia. The individual may speak in long sentences that have no meaning, add unnecessary words, and even create new words. They can make speech sounds; however, they have difficulty understanding speech and are therefore unaware of their mistakes.
- **Cortex:** is the surface of the cerebrum. It has a folded appearance with hills and valleys. The cortex contains 16 billion neurons (the cerebellum has 70 billion = 86 billion total) that are arranged in specific layers. The nerve cell bodies color the cortex grey-brown, giving it its name – gray matter (Figure 1.2(b)). Beneath the cortex are long nerve fibers (axons) that connect brain areas to each other, called white matter.

  The folding of the cortex increases the brain's surface area, allowing more neurons to fit inside the skull and enabling higher functions. Each fold is called a gyrus, and each groove between the folds is called a sulcus (Figure 1.2(b)). There are names for the folds and grooves that help define specific brain regions.

1.4.2 Deep Structures in the Brain and Their Functions

Pathways called white matter tracts connect areas of the cortex to each other. Messages can travel from one gyrus to another, from one lobe to another, from one side of the brain to the other, and to structures deep in the brain (Figure 1.2(b)).

- **Thalamus:** Ref Figure 1.3(a), serves as a relay station for almost all information that comes and goes to the cortex. It plays a role in pain sensation, attention, alertness, and memory.
- **Pituitary gland:** Ref Figure 1.3(a), lies in a small pocket of bone at the skull base called the sella turcica. The pituitary gland is connected to the hypothalamus of the brain by the pituitary stalk. Known as the "master gland," it controls other endocrine glands in the body. It secretes hormones that control sexual development, promote bone and muscle growth, and respond to stress.
- **Hypothalamus:** Ref Figure 1.3(a), is located in the floor of the third ventricle and is the master control of the autonomic system. It plays a role in controlling behaviors such as hunger, thirst, sleep, and sexual

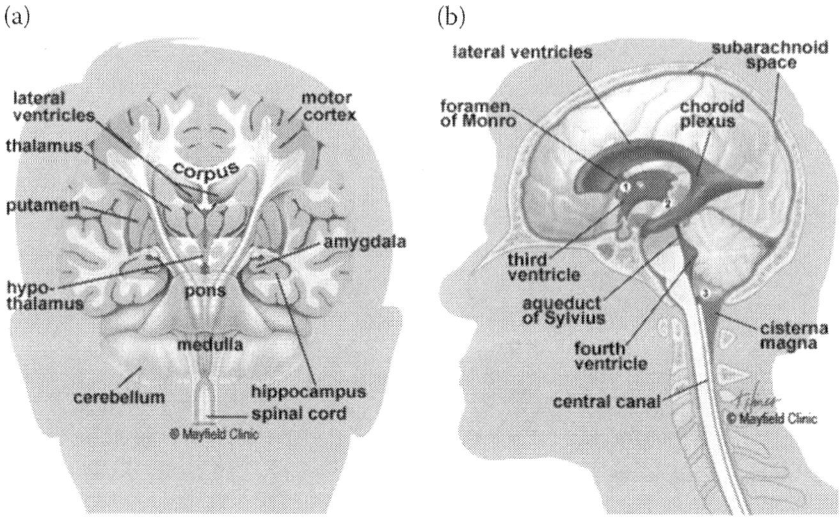

FIGURE 1.3 (a) Coronal cross-section showing the basal ganglia. (b) CSF is produced inside the ventricles deep within the brain. CSF fluid circulates inside the brain and spinal cord and then outside to the subarachnoid space.

response. It also regulates body temperature, blood pressure, emotions, and secretion of hormones.

- **Pineal gland:** is located behind the third ventricle. It helps regulate the body's internal clock and circadian rhythms by secreting melatonin. It has some role in sexual development.
- **Basal ganglia:** includes the caudate, putamen, and globus pallidus. These nuclei work with the cerebellum to coordinate fine motions, such as fingertip movements.
- **Limbic system:** is the center of our emotions, learning, and memory. Included in this system are the cingulate gyri, hypothalamus, amygdala (emotional reactions), and hippocampus (memory).

1.4.3 Memory

Memory is a complex process that includes three phases viz. encoding (deciding what information is important), storing, and recalling. Different areas of the brain are involved in different types of memory functions. Your brain has to pay attention and rehearse in order to port and move an event from short-term memory to long-term memory, which is called encoding.

- **Short-term memory**, also called working memory, occurs in the prefrontal cortex. It stores information for about one minute and its capacity is limited to about seven items. For example, it enables you to dial a phone number someone just told you. It also intervenes during reading, to memorize the sentence you have just read, so that the next one makes sense.

- **Long-term memory** is processed in the hippocampus of the temporal lobe and is activated when you want to memorize something for a longer time. This memory has unlimited content and duration capacity. It contains personal memories as well as facts and figures.
- **Skill memory** is processed in the cerebellum, which relays information to the basal ganglia. It stores automatic learned memories like tying a shoe, playing an instrument, or riding a bike.

1.4.4 Ventricles and Cerebrospinal Fluid

The brain has hollow fluid-filled cavities called ventricles (Figure 1.3(b)). Inside the ventricles is a ribbon-like structure called the choroid plexus that makes clear colorless cerebrospinal fluid (CSF). CSF flows within and around the brain and spinal cord to help cushion it from injury. This circulating fluid is constantly being absorbed and replenished.

There are two ventricles deep within the cerebral hemispheres called the lateral ventricles. They both connect with the third ventricle through a separate opening called the foramen of Monro. The third ventricle connects with the fourth ventricle through a long, narrow tube called the aqueduct of Sylvius. From the fourth ventricle, CSF flows into the subarachnoid space where it bathes and cushions the brain. CSF is recycled (or absorbed) by special structures in the superior sagittal sinus called arachnoid villi.

A balance is maintained between the amount of CSF that is absorbed and the amount that is produced. A disruption or blockage in the system can cause a buildup of CSF, which can cause enlargement of the ventricles (hydrocephalus) or cause a collection of fluid in the spinal cord (syringomyelia).

1.5 BRAIN CELLS AND THEIR COMMUNICATION MECHANISM

The brain is made up of two types of cells: nerve cells (neurons) and glia cells. These cells are the basic mechanism of communication within the brain. Together with synapse they form a network that is known as a neural network. A neural network has been modeled mathematically and implemented as computing algorithms in many different ways and form a major research area in computing science.

1.5.1 Nerve Cells

There are many sizes and shapes of neurons, but all consist of a cell body, dendrites, and an axon. The neuron conveys information through electrical and chemical signals. Try to picture electrical wiring in your home. An electrical circuit is made up of numerous wires connected in such a way that when a light switch is turned on, a lightbulb will beam. A neuron that is excited will transmit its energy to neurons within its vicinity.

Neurons transmit their energy, or "talk," to each other across a tiny gap called a synapse (Figure 1.4). A neuron has many arms called dendrites, which act like antennae picking up messages from other nerve cells. These messages are passed to the cell body, which determines if the message should be passed along. Important messages are passed to the end of the axon where sacs containing neurotransmitters open into the synapse. The neurotransmitter molecules cross the synapse and fit into special receptors on the receiving nerve cell, which stimulate that cell to pass on the message.

- **Glia cells:** Glia (Greek word meaning "glue") are the cells of the brain that provide neurons with nourishment, protection, and structural support. There are about 10 to 50 times more glia than nerve cells and are the most common type of cells involved in brain tumors.

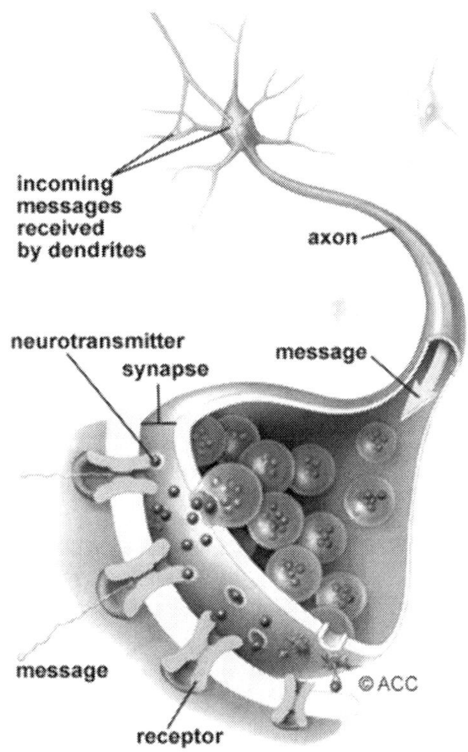

FIGURE 1.4 Nerve cells consist of a cell body, dendrites, and axon. Neurons communicate with each other by exchanging neurotransmitters across a tiny gap called a synapse.

- Astroglia or astrocytes are the caretakers – they regulate the blood brain barrier, allowing nutrients and molecules to interact with neurons. They control homeostasis, neuronal defense and repair, scar formation, and also affect electrical impulses.
- Oligodendroglia cells create a fatty substance called myelin that insulates axons – allowing electrical messages to travel faster.
- Ependymal cells line the ventricles and secrete cerebrospinal fluid (CSF).

Microglia are the brain's immune cells, protecting it from invaders and cleaning up debris. They also prune synapses.

1.6 NEUROIMAGING TECHNIQUES

Brain imaging techniques or neuroimaging techniques allow doctors and researchers to view activity or problems within the human brain, without invasive neurosurgery. There are a number of accepted, safe imaging techniques in use today in research facilities and hospitals throughout the world. Prominent brain imaging techniques that are available to cognitive neuroscientists, including positron emission tomography (PET), near infrared spectroscopy (NIRS), magnetoencephalogram (MEG), electroencephalography (EEG), and functional magnetic resonance imaging (fMRI). We discuss most of the available neuroimaging techniques in this section but focus on EEG and fMRI because they are the most widely used techniques.

1.6.1 Electroencephalography (EEG)

First discovered about a century ago, an EEG measures electrical activities of the brain from electrodes placed on the scalp. Usually, an EEG is collected from a number of electrodes positioned on different locations on the scalp. Most EEG systems used in cognitive neuroscience research today employ 64 to 256 electrodes. A scalp EEG represents the aggregates of post-synaptic currents of millions of neurons. The recorded EEG signals usually reflect two types of brain activities: *spontaneous* and *event-related activities*. A spontaneous EEG reflects neuronal responses that occur unprovoked, i.e., in the absence of any identifiable stimulus, with or without behavioral manifestations. A spontaneous EEG has long been used in clinical settings to evaluate seizure disorders, and now has been used often in cognitive neuroscience research.

1.6.2 Functional Magnetic Resonance Imaging (fMRI)

fMRI is one of the most recently developed forms of neuroimaging techniques. Since the early 1990s, fMRI has become the dominant method in cognitive neuroscience because of its low invasiveness, lack of radiation exposure, and relatively wide availability. In the brain, neural activities often lead to metabolic activities such as increased blood flow and oxygen supply to the local vasculature. Several variants of fMRI are used to detect changes of metabolic activities following neural activities, including *contrast fMRI*, *blood-oxygen-level dependent (BOLD) fMRI*, and *perfusion fMRI*. Contrast fMRI requires injection of contrast agents, such as iron oxide coated with sugar or starch. The signals associated with contrast agents are proportional to the cerebral blood volume (CBV). Although this method can provide relatively strong signals, researchers are reluctant to use this semi-invasive method with healthy volunteers. Perfusion fMRI uses "arterial spin labeling" (ASL) to magnetically label hydrogen nuclei in the arterial blood and then images their distribution in the brain. This method is sensitive to cerebral blood flow (CBF), which is considered a good correlate of neuronal activity. This method does not require any contrast agents. Compared to the BOLD responses, the signal in perfusion fMRI is more stable and the noise is much whiter. However, the relatively weak signal and the length of image acquisition time have limited the use of perfusion fMRI in cognitive neuroscience.

Currently, the most widely used fMRI method is BOLD imaging, which detects the difference in magnetic susceptibility between oxygenated hemoglobin and deoxygenated hemoglobin. Hemoglobin is diamagnetic when oxygenated but paramagnetic when deoxygenated. The magnetic property of blood therefore depends on its oxygenation level. Although neuronal activities consume some oxygen, the increase in blood flow following neuronal activities supplies more oxygen than the neuronal consumption, resulting in an increase in oxygenated hemoglobin and therefore increased BOLD response. Although BOLD fMRI is an indirect measure of neuronal activities, there is strong empirical evidence that the BOLD signals are highly correlated with neuronal activities. Because the BOLD signals are usually stronger and require less time to acquire than perfusion signals, BOLD fMRI is more popular than perfusion fMRI.

Other popular neuroimaging techniques practiced are as follows.

1.6.3 Computed Tomography (CT)

Computed tomography (CT) scanning builds up a picture of the brain based on the differential absorption of X-rays. During a CT scan the subject lies on a table that slides in and out of a hollow, cylindrical apparatus. An X-ray source rides on a ring around the inside of the tube, with its beam aimed at the subject's head. After passing through the head, the beam is sampled by one of the many detectors that line the machine's circumference. Images made using X-rays depend on the absorption of the beam by the tissue it passes through. Bone and hard tissue absorb X-rays well, air and water absorb very little, and soft tissue is somewhere in between. Thus, CT scans reveal the gross features of the brain but do not resolve its structure well.

1.6.4 Positron Emission Tomography (PET)

Positron emission tomography (PET) uses trace amounts of short-lived radioactive material to map functional processes in the brain. When the material undergoes radioactive decay, a positron is emitted, which can be picked up by the detector. Areas of high radioactivity are associated with brain activity.

1.6.5 Magnetoencephalography (MEG)

Magnetoencephalography (MEG) is an imaging technique used to measure the magnetic fields produced by electrical activity in the brain via extremely sensitive devices known as SQUIDs. These measurements are commonly used in both research and clinical settings. There are many uses for the MEG, including assisting surgeons in localizing a pathology, assisting researchers in determining the function of various parts of the brain, neurofeedback, and others.

1.6.6 Near Infrared Spectroscopy (NIRS)

Near infrared spectroscopy is an optical technique for measuring blood oxygenation in the brain. It works by shining light in the near infrared part of the spectrum (700–900 nm) through the skull and detecting how much the remerging light is attenuated. How much the light is attenuated depends on blood oxygenation and thus NIRS can provide an indirect measure of brain activity.

1.7 COMPARISON OF EEG AND FMRI

EEG and fMRI have their respective strengths and weaknesses. Ideally, experiments employing these methods must be carefully designed and conducted to maximize their strengths and minimize their weaknesses. The most salient feature of EEG is its high temporal resolution at a level of milliseconds. It is also a direct measure of neuronal response. Nevertheless, EEG has several limitations. First, EEG is only sensitive to post-synaptic potentials generated in the superficial layers of the cortex. It is not sensitive to neuronal responses from structures that are deep in the brain, such as the striatum or hippocampus. In addition, currents that are tangential to the skull make little contribution to the EEG signal. Second, the spatial resolution of EEG is very low. Third, it is almost impossible to reconstruct a unique intracranial current source distribution for a given EEG signal, although substantial recent progress has been made in this area.

In contrast, fMRI has high spatial resolution and a comprehensive coverage of the whole brain. Conventional BOLD fMRI has a typical spatial resolution of 3–6 mm; high-resolution fMRI can reach about 1 mm spatial resolution at the expense of whole-brain coverage. fMRI is sensitive to the BOLD signals from both the cortical surface and deep brain structures. The only limiting factor for coverage is susceptibility artifacts in the ventromedial prefrontal cortex and temporal poles. This problem has been partly resolved by some newly developed scanning sequences, or by using contrast fMRI and perfusion MRI. The major limitation of fMRI is its temporal resolution because the BOLD response is very slow. Moreover, the BOLD signal is only an indirect measure of neuronal activity, and is therefore susceptible to influence by many physiological activities of the body that are unrelated to neuronal processes.

1.8 ELECTROENCEPHALOGRAPHY (EEG)

Any synaptic activity generates a subtle electrical impulse referred to as a postsynaptic potential. It is difficult to reliably detect the burst of a single neuron without direct contact with it. However, whenever thousands of neurons fire in sync, they generate an electrical field thatis strong enough to spread through tissue, bone, and skull. Eventually, it can be measured on the surface of the head. This electrical signal is called as electroencephalography (EEG) signal.

Electroencephalography (EEG) is the physiological method to record the electrical activity generated by the brain. EEG is measured through electrodes placed on the surface of the scalp. For faster application, electrodes are mounted in elastic caps similar to bathing caps, ensuring that the data can be collected from identical scalp positions across all respondents.

Figure 1.5(a) describes the placement of electrodes on the scalp for EEG recording; 10–20 electrode placements are used for the experiments and out of these recordings the data corresponding to four channels of EEG data are plotted, as depicted in Figure 1.5(b).

The EEG signal is classified based on its frequency, amplitude, and phase. The physical characteristic of the EEG signal is classified as delta (δ), theta (Θ), alpha (α), beta (β), or gamma (γ).

Yet another way of defining an EEG is that the EEG measures voltage fluctuations resulting from ionic current within the neurons of the brain. Clinically, an EEG refers to the recording of the brain's spontaneous electrical activity over a period of time, as recorded from multiple electrodes placed on the scalp (Niedermeyer & da Silva 2004).

1.9 CLASSIFICATION OF EEG SIGNALS BASED ON FREQUENCIES

The frequency and voltage of an EEG signal generally varies from 1–50 Hz and 10–100 μV when measured from the skull surface. The EEG signal is classified according to range of frequency and voltage. In order of lowest frequency to highest, the five brain waves are: delta (δ), theta (Θ), alpha (α), beta (β), and gamma (γ) (Figure 1.6).

1.9.1 Delta Waves

Delta waves are associated with deep levels of relaxation and restorative sleeps; to remember this, simply think of "delta" for "deep." They are the slowest

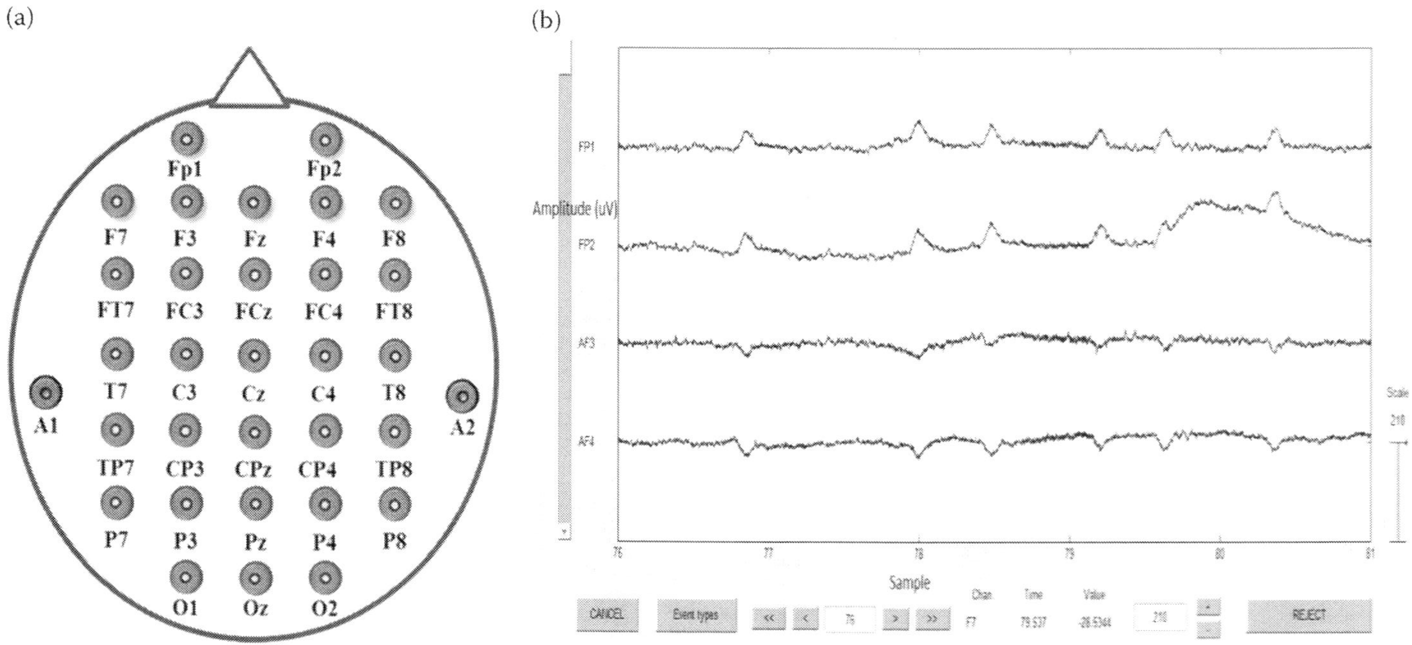

FIGURE 1.5 Electroencephalography (EEG) signal capture. (a) Placement of 10–20 electrodes for 32 channel EEG acquisition system. (b) Plot for EEG data from FP1, FP2, A1, A2 channel.

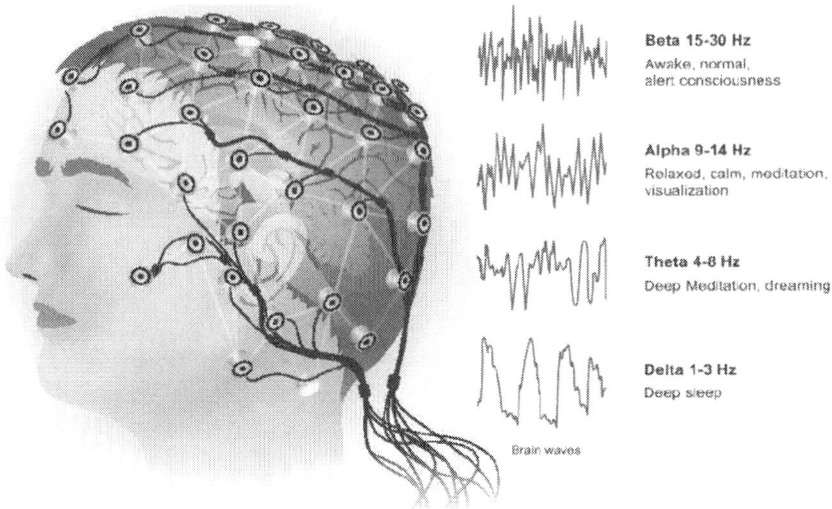

FIGURE 1.6 Classification of EEG waves.

recorded brain waves in humans and higher levels are more commonly found in young children. During the aging process, lower delta waves are produced. Research tells us that delta waves are attributed to many of our unconscious bodily functions such as regulating the cardiovascular and the digestive systems. Healthy levels of delta waves can contribute to a more restful sleep, allowing us to wake up refreshed; however, irregular delta wave activity has been linked to learning difficulties or issues maintaining awareness.

- **Frequency range:** 0 Hz to 4 Hz
- **High levels:** Brain injuries, learning problems, inability to think
- **Low levels:** Inability to rejuvenate body, inability to revitalize the brain, poor sleep or sleep disorder
- **Optimal range:** Healthy immune system, restorative REM sleep

1.9.2 Theta Waves

Theta waves are known as the "suggestible waves," because of their prevalence when one is in a trance or hypnotic state. In this state, a brain's theta waves are optimal and the patient is more susceptible to hypnosis and associated therapy. The reasoning for this is that theta waves are commonly found when you day-dream or are asleep, thus exhibiting a more relaxed, open mind state. Theta waves are also linked to us experiencing and feeling deep and raw emotions; therefore, too much theta activity may make people prone to bouts of depression. Theta does however have its benefits of helping improve our creativity, wholeness, and intuition, making us feel more natural. It is also involved in restorative sleep and as long as theta isn't produced in excess during our waking hours, it is a very helpful brainwave range.

- **Frequency range:** 4 Hz to 8 Hz
- **High levels:** ADHD or hyperactivity, depressive states, impulsive activity or inattentiveness
- **Low levels:** Anxiety symptoms, poor emotional awareness, higher stress levels
- **Optimal range:** Maximum creativity, deep emotional connection with oneself and others, greater intuition, relaxation

1.9.3 Alpha Waves

Alpha waves are the "frequency bridge" between our conscious thinking (beta) and subconscious (theta) mind. They are known to help calm you down and promote feelings of deeper relaxation and content. Beta waves play an active role in network coordination and communication and do not occur until three years of age in humans. In a state of stress, a phenomenon called "alpha blocking" can occur, which involves excessive beta activity and little alpha activity. In this scenario, the beta waves restrict the production of alpha because our body is reacting positively to the increased beta activity, usually in a state of heightened cognitive arousal.

- **Frequency range:** 8 Hz to 12 Hz
- **High levels:** Too much daydreaming, over-relaxed state or an inability to focus
- **Low levels:** OCD, anxiety symptoms, higher stress levels
- **Optimal range:** Ideal relaxation

1.9.4 Beta Waves

Beta waves are the high-frequency waves most commonly found in the awake state of humans. They are channeled during conscious states such as cognitive reasoning, calculation, reading, speaking, or thinking. Higher levels of beta waves are found to channel a stimulating, arousing effect, which explains how the brain will limit the amount of alpha waves if heightened beta activity occurs. However, if you experience too much beta activity, this may lead to stress and anxiety. This leads you to feel overwhelmed and stressed during strenuous periods of work or school. Beta waves increased by drinking common stimulants such as caffeine or L-Theanine, or by consuming nootropics or cognitive enhancers such as lucid. Think of beta as the stressed state of mind.

- **Frequency range:** 12 Hz to 40 Hz
- **High levels:** Anxiety, inability to feel relaxed, high adrenaline levels, stress, cognitive actions

- **Low levels:** Depression, poor cognitive ability, lack of attention
- **Optimal range:** Consistent focus, strong memory recall, high problem-solving ability

1.9.5 Gamma Waves

Gamma waves are a more recent discovery in the field of neuroscience; thus, the understanding of how they function is constantly evolving. To date, it's known that gamma waves are involved in processing more complex tasks in addition to healthy cognitive function. Gamma waves are found to be important for learning, memory, and processing and they are used as a binding tool for our senses to process new information. In people with mental disabilities, much lower levels of gamma activity are recorded. More recently, people have found a strong link between meditation and gamma waves, a link attributed to the heightened state of being or "completeness" experienced when in a meditative state.

- **Frequency range:** Above 40 Hz
- **High levels:** Anxiety, stress
- **Low levels:** Depression, learning issues, diagnosis of ADHD (brain scientists have found that deficiencies in specific neurotransmitters underlie many common disorders, including anxiety, mood disorders, anger-control problems, and obsessive-compulsive disorder). ADHD was the first disorder found to be the result of a deficiency of a specific neurotransmitter.
- **Optimal range:** Information processing, cognition, learning, binding of senses.

For ease of reading, the classification of different bands of EEG signals are shown in Table 1.1.

TABLE 1.1
EEG classification according to frequency

Sl No.	Type	Frequency (Hz)	State of Mind
1	Delta	0–4	Healthy immune system, restorative REM sleep
2	Theta	4–8	Maximum creativity, deep emotional connection with oneself and others, greater intuition, relaxation
3	Alpha	8–12	Ideal relaxation
4	Beta	12–40	Consistent focus, strong memory recall, high problem-solving ability
5	Gamma	Above 40	Information processing, cognition, learning, binding of senses

1.10 ELECTROOCULOGRAPHY (EOG)

Electrooculography (EOG) is used to record eye movements during electronystagmographic testing. It is based on the corneo-retinal potential (difference in electrical charge between the cornea and the retina), with the long axis of the eye acting as a dipole. This potential is thought to result from the metabolic activity of the retina. When the eye rotates in the orbit, the dipole also rotates. Silver–silver chloride electrodes placed near the orbit can be used to record this electrical difference. To measure eye movement, pairs of electrodes are typically placed either above and below the eye or to the left and right of the eye. If the eye moves from center position toward one of the two electrodes, this electrode "sees" the positive side of the retina and the opposite electrode "sees" the negative side of the retina. Consequently, a potential difference occurs between the electrodes. Assuming that the resting potential is constant, the recorded potential is a measure of the eye's position.

In other words, a record of the standing voltage between the front and back of the eye that is correlated with eyeball movement (as in REM sleep) and obtained by electrodes suitably placed on the skin near the eye is called EOG. Electrooculography was used by Robert Zemeckis and Jerome Chen, the visual effects supervisors in the movie *Beowulf*, to enhance the performance capture by correctly animating the eye movements of the actors. The result was an improvement over the technique used for the film *The Polar Express*. Some of the key applications of EOG are as follows:

- EOG can be used to detect eye movement and related artifacts. Blink, saccade, and fix are three major artifacts that can be analyzed from EOG.
- Blink artifacts are considered as noise to the signal; therefore, filtering those result in more accurate experimental information to analyze further (Kong & Wilson 1998). Blink detection can also be used for drowsiness detection, attention analysis, etc.
- Saccade are voltage deflection when the eye moves randomly from one fix to another.

1.11 APPLICATIONS OF EEG

The genesis of EEG is attributed to the diagnostic need in medical science for better understanding of the dynamics of the human brain. Because of its growing utility in different domains, EEG has emerged as a field of collaboration with many emerging sciences and technologies. Therefore, it is apt to describe this collaborative nature through a mapping of all the associated science, technology, system, and associated applications in the form of concept mapping of EEG. Figure 1.7 describes an approximate concept mapping of EEG and its emerging applications.

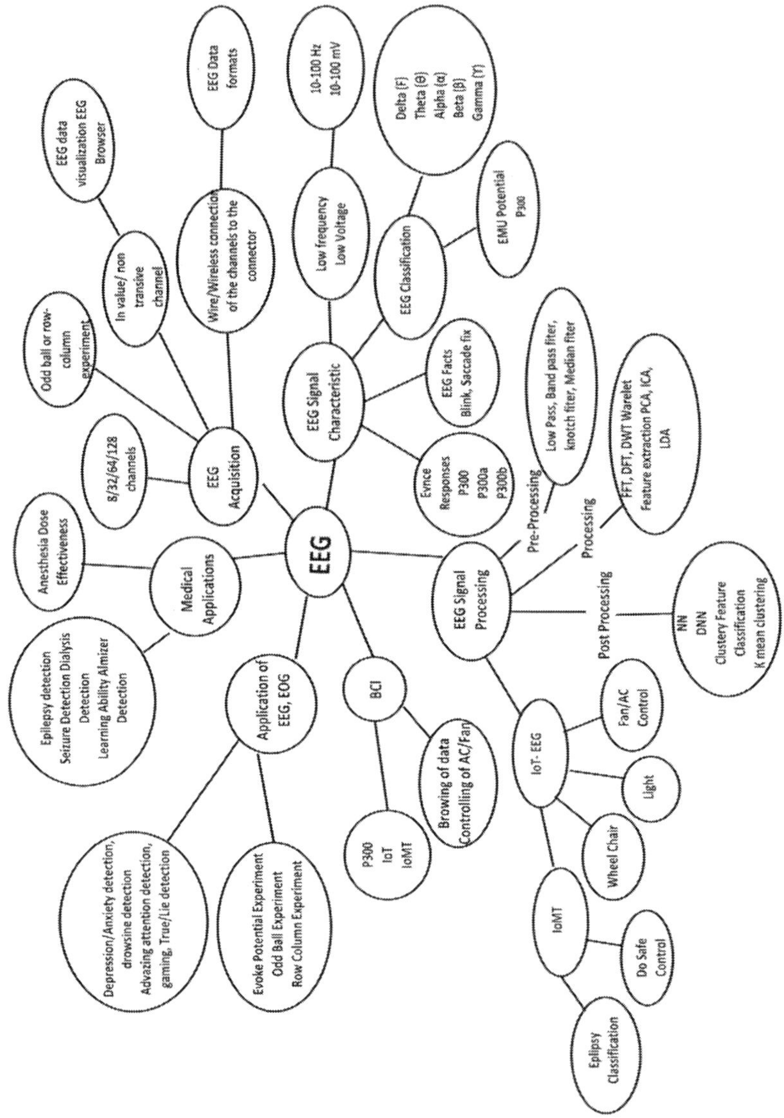

FIGURE 1.7 Mind mapping of concepts and applications of EEG.

EEG has given way to many areas of new research and applications besides its traditional application in medicine. Some emerging applications are in the field of BCI, neuro-marketing, cognitive capacity building, and therapy, etc. Some of the key applications of EEG are described.

1.11.1 Medical Applications

- The EEG is used to evaluate several types of brain disorders. When epilepsy is present, seizure activity will appear as rapid spiking waves on the EEG.
- People with lesions on their brain (i.e., *brain lesions* (*lesions* on the *brain*) refers to any type of abnormal tissue in or on the brain tissue). Major types of *brain lesions* are traumatic, infectious, malignant, benign, vascular, genetic, immune, plaques, *brain* cell death or malfunction, and ionizing radiation, which can result from tumors or strokes, and may have unusually slow EEG waves, depending on the size and the location of the lesion.
- The test can also be used to diagnose other disorders that influence brain activity, such as Alzheimer's disease, certain psychoses, and a sleep disorder called narcolepsy (Farnsworth 2020).

1.11.2 Commercial Applications

- In the field of neuro-marketing, economists use EEG research to detect brain processes that drive consumer decisions, brain areas that are active when we purchase a product/service, and mental states that the respective person is in when exploring physical or virtual stores. (Electroencephalogram (EEG) 2020; Sebastian 2014).

1.12 BRAIN COMPUTER INTERFACE (BCI)

A brain computer interface (BCI) is a computer-based system that requires brain signals, analyzes them, and translates them into commands that are relayed to an output device to carry out a desired action. In principle, any brain signal could be used to control the BCI, but an EEG signal is used in most of the BCI systems because the EEG is an non-invasive signal acquisition method. The EEG signal corresponding to any spatial portion of the brain identified by its corresponding electrode can be analyzed, leading a direct functional interpretation of the brain signal. Also, the cost of EEG acquisition is substantially less in comparison to other brain-signal acquisition techniques. Classification of BCI systems based on prevailing neuroimaging systems is given in Figure 1.8. Some of the popular applications of BCI are as follows:

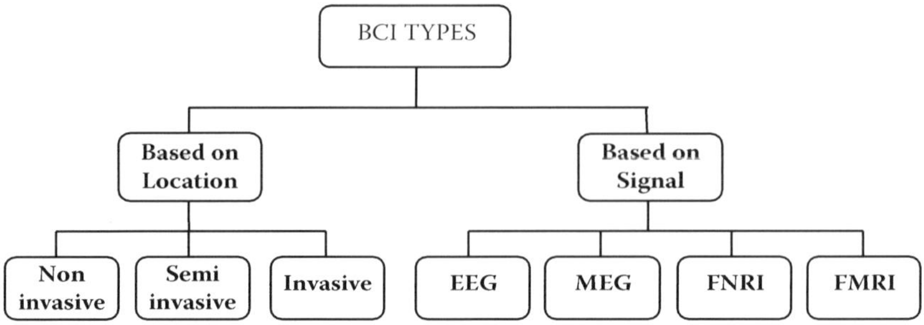

FIGURE 1.8 Different types of brain computer interface BCI.

- Analyze EEG signals of paralyzed patients and provide them a degree of independence for certain tasks like home-based application control (Bastiaansen et al 2018), wheelchair control (Srivastava et al 2015), etc.
- EEG-based assistive mobile robots (Maksud et al 2017; Chae et al 2012).
- Measure a person's cognitive ability and improvement in cognitive functions (Akhanda et al 2014; Mora Sanchez et al 2015).

1.13 SUMMARY

This chapter first gives an overview of the anatomy of the human brain, with a perspective to look into its various functions. An overview of different neuroimaging techniques were discussed with an emphasis on the most popular neuroimaging methods: EEG and fMRI. The applications of various neuroimaging techniques in research were looked into. The EEG signal can be very useful for BCI applications because of its high spatial and temporal resolution, capturing the details of neuroimaging functions. That is why EEG processing is finding favor among different domains such as health care, IOT, virtual reality, and psychological study. It can also be used for driver/pilot assistance by performing drowsiness and consciousness detection. A classification of various components present in EEG signals, their signal and voltage characteristics, along with possible physical interpretation of the state of the brain was discussed. The main constraint with an EEG signal is that it is low in signal strength and low on signal frequency as well. A lot of pre-processing is required to boost the signal, which may include noise. In later chapters, we discuss about various pre-processing and post-processing techniques suitable for bringing out different features from the EEG signal.

Exercises

1. What are different functional parts of the human brain?
2. Give a diagrammatic representation of a nerve cell and list its functions.

3. Give a brief mapping of different functional lobes present in the brain. Give a brief mapping of different functions governed by these lobes.
4. List different neuroimaging techniques and their research applications.
5. What is an EEG? What are different characteristic signals present in an EEG?
6. Write a short note on EEG and fMRI and compare and contrast EEG and fMRI.
7. What are the different types of EEG signals? List their signal characteristic and physical manifestations.
8. What is EOG? How is EOG useful?
9. Give different configurations of EEG acquisition systems.
10. List some of medical and diagnostic applications of EEG.
11. Give a classification of various neuroimaging techniques.
12. What is a brain computer interface? List five popular applications of BCI.

REFERENCES

Akhanda, MABS, Islam, SMF & Rahman, MM 2014, 'Detection of cognitive state for brain-computer interfaces', in *2013 International Conference on Electrical Information and Communication Technology (EICT)*, Khulna, pp. 1–6. doi:10.1109/EICT.2014.6777878

Apps, R & Garwicz, M 2005, 'Anatomical and physiological foundations of cerebellar information processing', *Nature Reviews Neuroscience*, vol. 6, no. 4, pp. 297–311. PMID 15803161. doi:10.1038/nrn1646

Bastiaansen, M, Straatman, S & Driessen, E 2018, 'OndrejMitas, JeroenStekelenburg, Lin Wang, My destination in your brain: A novel neuromarketing approach for evaluating the effectiveness of destination marketing', *Journal of Destination Marketing & Management*, vol. 7, pp. 76–88. ISSN 2212-571X. doi:10.1016/j.jdmm.2016.09.003

Chae, Y, Jeong, J & Jo, S 2012, 'Toward brain-actuated humanoid robots: Asynchronous direct-control using an EEG-based BCI', *IEEE Transactions on Robotics*, vol. 28, pp. 1131–1144. doi:10.1109/TRO.2012.2201310

Electroencephalogram (EEG), https://www.hopkinsmedicine.org/health/treatment-tests-and-therapies/electroencephalogram-eeg, Last Accessed on 27 June 2020.

Farnsworth, B 2020 June, *What is EEG (Electroencephalography) and How Does it Work?*, https://imotions.com/blog/what-is-eeg/, Last Accessed on 27 June 2020.

Kong, X & Wilson, GF 1998, 'A new EOG-based eyeblink detection algorithm', *Behaviour Research Methods, Instruments, & Computers: A Journal of the Psychonomic Society, Inc.*, vol. 30, pp. 713–719. doi:10.3758/BF03209491

Maksud, A, Chowdhury, RI, Chowdhury, TT, Fattah, SA, Shahanaz, C & Chowdhury, SS 2017, 'Low-cost EEG based electric wheelchair with advanced control features', in *TENCON 2017 – 2017 IEEE Region 10 Conference*, Penang, pp. 2648–2653. doi:10.1109/TENCON.2017.8228309.

Mora Sanchez, A, Gaume, A, Dreyfus, G & Vialatte, F 2015, 'A cognitive brain-computer interface prototype for the continuous monitoring of visual working memory load', IEEE 25th International Workshop on Machine Learning for Signal Processing (MLSP), IEEE: Boston, MA, USA, doi:10.1109/MLSP.2015.732437

Niedermeyer, E & da Silva, FL 2004, *Electroencephalography: Basic Principles, Clinical Applications, and Related Fields*. Lippincott Williams & Wilkins. ISBN 978-0-7817-5126-1.

Sebastian, V 2014, 'Neuromarketing and evaluation of cognitive and emotional responses of consumers to marketing stimuli', *Procedia – Social and Behavioral Sciences*, vol. 127, pp. 753–757. ISSN 1877-0428. doi:10.1016/j.sbspro.2014.03.349

Srivastava, A, Lal, M, Jain, D, Furkan, M & Singh, A January 2015, 'EEG based home appliance control for providing guidance to paralyzed person', *International Journal of Electrical, Electronics and Data Communication*, vol. 3, no. 1, pp. 23–26. ISSN 2320-2084.

2 Fundamentals of EEG Signals

2.1 INTRODUCTION

The EEG represents the electrical activity of the cerebral cortex originating from the sum of excitatory and inhibitory postsynaptic activity in the brain. The EEG is regulated by the sub-cortical thalamic nuclei. This electrical signal has direct relevance to physical activities controlled by different parts of the brain. Cerebral blood flow and brain metabolism are directly related to the degree or magnitude of the EEG signal. When patients are unconscious and unresponsive, the EEG is a non-invasive indicator of brain function. Recording an unprocessed raw EEG involves accumulation of large amounts of EEG records and storage in a computer memory. Different computing techniques have been devised to analyze and map these EEG signals to extract meaningful information. Also, various functions of the brain can be correlated to different physical manifestations through study and analysis of EEG signals.

Recently, several signal processing techniques have been devised to better analyze different fundamental patterns in the EEG. The purpose of these techniques and signal processing technologies is to simplify and analyze the EEG for use in various fields such as diagnosis of dyslexia, neurological disease, seizure, and to devise a brain computer interface. Many statistical properties associated with the EEG signal can be correlated to different functional and diagnostic aspects.

The EEG is a complex signal that represents the electrical activity of the brain. Like other signals, the EEG can also be split into a series of sinusoids. In some analyses, the EEG parameters are processed based on power spectral analysis. Power spectral analysis considers the amplitude of sinusoids as a function of frequency. However, power spectral analysis does not quantify the possible relationships between sinusoids. Such relationships between these elements typically appear in signals generated in nonlinear systems such as the brain. Power spectral analysis of the EEG clearly ignores the relationship between sinusoids. Almost all biological systems and EEGs show considerably nonlinear behavior. Because of the nonlinear characteristics of neuronal activity, the EEG signal has very complex dynamics. An analytical technique that can detect and quantify any aspect of this nonlinear change may better reflect the dynamic structure of the EEG. Here, the basic elements and terminology of signal processing, followed by Fourier analysis and power spectrum analysis, were briefly discussed.

DOI: 10.1201/9781003241386-2

2.2 MODELING OF EEG SIGNALS

One of the earliest physical models of an EEG signal was proposed by Hodgkin and Huxley, who eventually were awarded a Nobel Prize. Most of the current neural network simulations and computational neuroscience findings are based on Hodgkin and Huxley's physical model. Therefore, it is worthwhile to discuss and understand this model. This model was for the squid axon published in 1952 (Hodgkin & Huxley 1952a, 1952b, 1952c, 1952d; Hodgkin et al 1952). As per this theory, a nerve axon may be stimulated and activated by sodium (Na^+) and potassium (K^+) channels produced in the vicinity of the cell membrane that lead to the electrical excitation of the nerve axon. The excitation arises from the effect of the membrane potential on the movement of ions, and from interactions of the membrane potential with the opening and closing of voltage-activated membrane channels. The membrane potential increases when the membrane is polarized with a net negative charge lining on the inner surface and an equal but opposite net positive charge on the outer surface. This potential can be related to the amount of electrical charge Q, which is described using Equation 2.1:

$$E = Q/C_m \tag{2.1}$$

where Q is in terms of coulombs/cm^2, C_m is the measure of the capacity of the membrane in units of farads/cm^2, and E is in units of volts.

In practice, in order to model the action potentials (APs), the amount of charge Q^+ on the inner surface and Q^- on the outer surface of the cell membrane has to be mathematically related to the stimulating current I_{stim} flowing into the cell through the stimulating electrodes. The electrical potential (often called the electrical force) E is then calculated using Equation 2.1. Hodgkin and Huxley's model is illustrated in Figure 2.1. In this figure, I_{memb} is the result of positive charges flowing out of the cell. This current consists of three currents: Na, K, and leak currents. The leak current is due to the fact that the inner and outer Na and K ions are not exactly equal.

Hodgkin and Huxley estimated the activation and inactivation functions for the Na and K currents and derived a mathematical model to describe an AP similar to that of a giant squid. The model is a neuron model that uses voltage-gated channels. The space-clamped version of the Hodgkin–Huxley model can be well described using four ordinary differential equations (Hodgkin et al 1952). This model describes the change in the membrane potential (E) with respect to time (Hodgkin & Huxley 1952d). The overall membrane current is the sum of capacity current and ionic current, as described in Equation 2.2:

$$I_{memb} = C_m \frac{dE}{dt} + I_i \tag{2.2}$$

where I_i is the ionic current and, as indicated in Figure 2.1. It can be considered as the sum of three individual components, Na, K, and leak currents, as given by Equation 2.3:

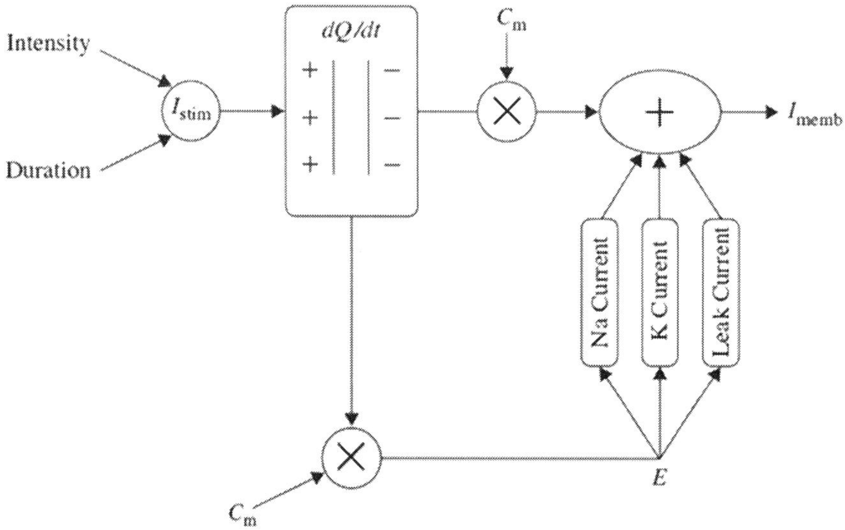

FIGURE 2.1 The Hodgkin–Huxley excitation model for the generation of action potentials.

$$I_i = I_{Na} + I_K + I_{leak} \tag{2.3}$$

Further, the individual components in Equation 2.3, such as I_{Na}, can be related to the maximal conductance $\bar{g}_{Na}$, activation variable a_{Na}, inactivation variable h_{Na}, and a driving force $(E - E_{Na})$ which is modeled in Equation 2.4:

$$I_{Na} = \bar{g}_{Na} a_{Na}^3 h_{Na} (E - E_{Na}) \tag{2.4}$$

Similarly, I_K can be related to the maximal conductance $\bar{g}_K$, activation variable a_{Na}, inactivation variable a_K, and a driving force $(E - E_K)$, which is modeled in Equation 2.5:

$$I_K = \bar{g}_K a_K (E - E_K) \tag{2.5}$$

and I_{leak} is related to the maximal conductance $\bar{g}_l$ and a driving force $(E - E_l)$, which is given by Equation 2.6:

$$I_l = \bar{g}_l (E - E_l) \tag{2.6}$$

The changes in the variables, a_{Na}, a_K, and h_{Na}, vary from 0–1 and are modeled as per Equations 2.7, 2.8, and 2.9, given below:

$$\frac{da_{\text{Na}}}{dt} = \lambda_t \left[\alpha_{\text{Na}}(E)(1 - a_{\text{Na}}) - \beta_{\text{Na}}(E) a_{\text{Na}} \right] \tag{2.7}$$

$$\frac{dh_{\text{Na}}}{dt} = \lambda_t \left[\alpha_{\text{h}}(E)(1 - h_{\text{Na}}) - \beta_{\text{h}}(E) h_{\text{Na}} \right] \tag{2.8}$$

$$\frac{da_{\text{K}}}{dt} = \lambda_t \left[\alpha_{\text{K}}(E)(1 - a_{\text{K}}) - \beta_{\text{K}}(E) a_{\text{K}} \right] \tag{2.9}$$

where $\alpha(E)$ and $\beta(E)$ are respectively forward and backward rate functions and λ_t is a temperature-dependent factor. The forward and backward parameters depend on voltage and were empirically estimated by Hodgkin and Huxley through Equations 2.10–2.15:

$$\alpha_{\text{Na}}(E) = \frac{3.5 + 0.1E}{1 - e^{-(3.5+0.1E)}} \tag{2.10}$$

$$\beta_{\text{Na}}(E) = 4e^{-(E+60)/18} \tag{2.11}$$

$$\alpha_{\text{h}}(E) = 0.07e^{-(E+60)/20} \tag{2.12}$$

$$\beta_{\text{h}}(E) = \frac{1}{1 + e^{-(3+0.1E)}} \tag{2.13}$$

$$\alpha_{\text{K}}(E) = \frac{0.5 + 0.01E}{1 - e^{-(5+0.1E)}} \tag{2.14}$$

$$\beta_{\text{K}}(E) = 0.125e^{-(E+60)/80} \tag{2.15}$$

As stated in the simulator for neural networks and action potentials (SNNAP) literature (Hodgkin & Huxley 1952d), the $\alpha(E)$ and $\beta(E)$ parameters have been converted from the original Hodgkin–Huxley version to agree with the present physiological practice, where depolarization of the membrane is taken to be positive. In addition, the resting potential has been shifted to –60 mV (from the original 0 mV). These equations are used in the model described in the SNNAP. In Figure 2.2, an AP has been simulated. For this model, the parameters are set to $C_{\text{m}} = 1.1\ \mu\text{F/cm}^2$, $\bar{g}_{\text{K}} = 100\ \text{ms/cm}^2$, $\bar{g}_{\text{K}} = 35\ \text{ms/cm}^2$, $\bar{g}_{\text{l}} = 0.35\ \text{ms/cm}^2$, and $E_{\text{Na}} = 60$ mV.

A simpler model than that due to Hodgkin–Huxley for simulating spiking neurons is the Morris–Lecar model (Forrest 2014). This model is a minimal

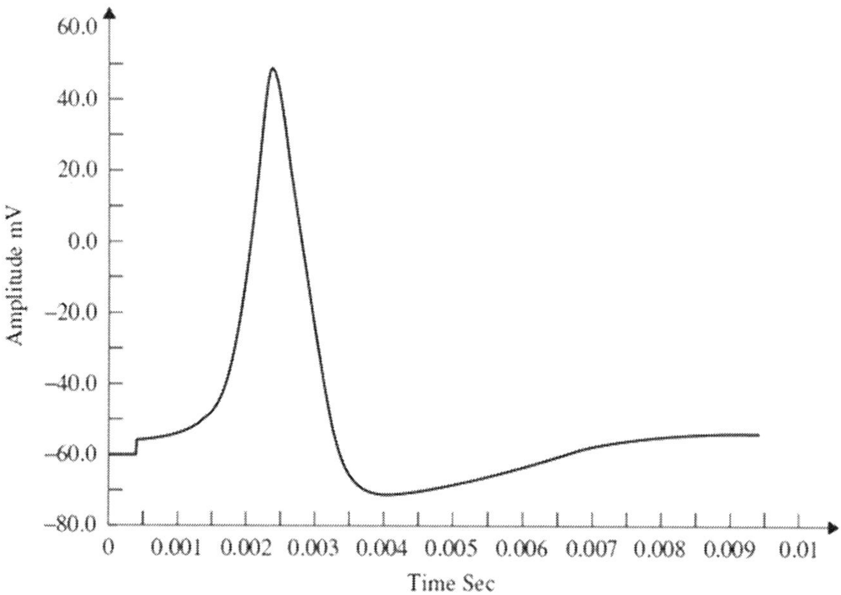

FIGURE 2.2 The voltage vs time plot of the EEG Hodgkin–Huxley oscillatory model.

biophysical model, which generally exhibits a single action potential. This model considers that the oscillation of a slow calcium wave that depolarizes the membrane leads to a bursting state. The Morris–Lecar model was initially developed to describe the behavior of barnacle muscle cells.

The plot of the EEG signal is (amplitude of EEG signal vs time) modeled using the Hodgkin–Huxley model, which is illustrated in Figure 2.2.

2.3 THE GENERAL CHARACTERISTICS OF EEG SIGNALS

Having discussed the modeling of EEG signal, this section discusses the characteristics of an EEG electrical signals (Figure 2.3), including how this analog signal is digitized and converted to a digital signal and how the digital EEG signal is formed from different known patterns or constituent signals. The electroencephalogram (EEG) is a recording of the electrical activity of the brain from the scalp. The recorded waveforms reflect the cortical electrical activity. The fundamental characteristics of human EEG signals include the following:

- **Signal Intensity:** EEG activity is quite small, measured in microvolts (1~100 μV).
- **Signal Frequency:** the main frequencies of the human EEG waves include the following:
    - **Delta**: has a frequency of 3 Hz or below. It tends to be the highest in amplitude and the slowest waves. It is normal as the dominant

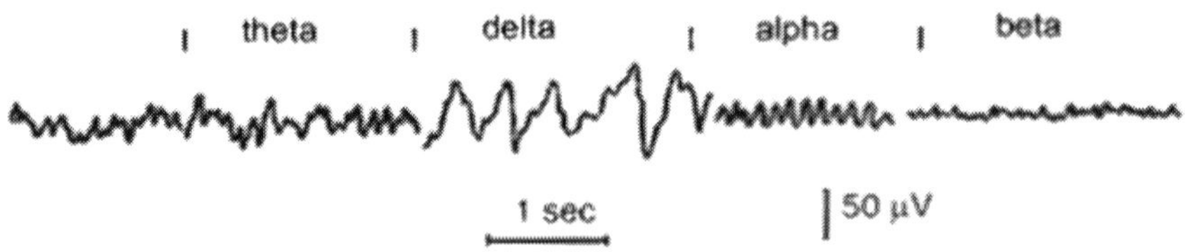

FIGURE 2.3 Patterns of different types of EEG signals.

rhythm in infants up to one year and in stages 3 and 4 of sleep. It may occur focally with subcortical lesions and in general distribution with diffuse lesions, metabolic encephalopathy hydrocephalus, or deep midline lesions. It is usually most prominent frontally in adults (e.g., FIRDA – Frontal Intermittent Rhythmic Delta) and posteriorly in children e.g., OIRDA – Occipital Intermittent Rhythmic Delta).

- **Theta**: has a frequency of 3.5 to 7.5 Hz and is classified as "slow" activity. It is perfectly normal in children up to 13 years and in sleep but abnormal in awake adults. It can be seen as a manifestation of focal subcortical lesions; it can also be seen in generalized distribution in diffuse disorders such as metabolic encephalopathy or some instances of hydrocephalus.
- **Alpha**: has a frequency between 7.5 and 13 Hz. It is usually best seen in the posterior regions of the head on each side, being higher in amplitude on the dominant side. It appears when closing the eyes and relaxing, and disappears when opening the eyes or alerted by any mechanism (thinking, calculating). It is the major rhythm seen in normal relaxed adults. It is present during most life, especially after the 13th year.
- **Beta**: beta activity is "fast" activity. It has a frequency of 14 and greater Hz. It is usually seen on both sides in symmetrical distribution and is most evident frontally. It is accentuated by sedative-hypnotic drugs, especially the benzodiazepines and the barbiturates. It may be absent or reduced in areas of cortical damage. It is generally regarded as a normal rhythm. It is the dominant rhythm in patients who are alert or anxious or have their eyes open.

2.4 ATTRIBUTES USED IN THE CLASSIFICATION OF EEG SIGNALS

Five fundamental attributes of EEG signals that are useful to completely describe the characteristics of EEG signal are (1) frequency, (2) voltage, (3) morphology, (4) synchrony, and (5) periodicity. One or a combination of the fundamental attributes are used to classify the EEG signal into the fundamental EEG waves of delta, theta, alpha, beta, and gamma types of activities. The EEG attributes are discussed below.

2.4.1 Frequency

EEG frequency refers to rhythmic, repetitive activity (in Hz). The frequency of EEG activity can have different properties including:

- **Rhythmic**: EEG activity consisting of waves of approximately constant frequency.
- **Arrhythmic**: EEG activity in which no stable rhythms are present.
- **Dysrhythmic**: Rhythms and/or patterns of EEG activity that characteristically appear in patient groups or are rarely seen in healthy subjects.

2.4.2 Voltage

Voltage refers to the average voltage or peak voltage of EEG activity. Values are dependent, in part, on the recording technique. Descriptive terms associated with EEG voltage include:

1. **Attenuation** (synonyms: suppression, depression). Reduction of amplitude of EEG activity resulting from decreased voltage. When activity is attenuated by stimulation, it is said to have been "blocked" or to show "blocking."
2. **Hypersynchrony**. Seen as an increase in voltage and regularity of rhythmic activity, or within the alpha, beta, or theta range. The term implies an increase in the number of neural elements contributing to the rhythm. (Note: Term is used in an interpretative sense but as a descriptor of change in the EEG.)
3. **Paroxysmal**. Activity that emerges from background with a rapid onset, reaching (usually) quite high voltage and ending with an abrupt return to lower voltage activity. Though the term does not directly imply abnormality, much abnormal activity is paroxysmal.

2.4.3 Morphology

Morphology refers to the shape of the waveform. The shape of a wave or an EEG pattern is determined by the frequencies that combine to make up the waveform and by their phase and voltage relationships. Wave patterns can be described as being:

- **Monomorphic**. Distinct EEG activity appearing to be composed of one dominant activity.

- **Polymorphic**. Distinct EEG activity composed of multiple frequencies that combine to form a complex waveform.
- **Sinusoidal**. Waves resembling sine waves; which represents monomorphic activity usually is sinusoidal.
- **Transient**. An isolated wave or pattern that is distinctly different from background activity.
  a. Spike: a transient with a pointed peak and a duration from 20 to under 70 msec.
  b. Sharp wave: a transient with a pointed peak and duration of 70–200 msec.

2.4.4 Synchrony

Synchrony refers to the simultaneous appearance of rhythmic or morphologically distinct patterns over different regions of the head, either on the same side (unilateral) or both sides (bilateral).

2.4.5 Periodicity

Periodicity refers to the distribution of patterns or elements in time (e.g., the appearance of a particular EEG activity at more or less regular intervals). The activity may be generalized, focal, or lateralized.

2.5 EEG SIGNALS AND SAMPLING

An EEG is a series of continuous analog electrical signals in time x(t). The process of converting an analog signal to a digital signal is called sampling or digitization of the signal. For example, if the time interval between samples is Δt and the number of samples in a particular segment in the collected data is M, then successive samples of the EEG signal x(t) can be denoted by x(k·Δt), where k = 0, 1, 2, …, M−1. These sample values of the EEG signal x(t) in time instances 0·Δt, 1·Δt, 2·Δt, … (M−1)·Δt are called the digitized value of the sample. The entire sampled EEG data can be represented by $x(k)$, and x(k) can be divided into a series of sequential epochs (same time segments). These epochs may overlap each other or be contiguous.

If the statistical characteristics of the signal do not change with time, the signal is called stationary. The stationary signal can be represented by the sum of simple mathematical functions (elements) and all information of the signal can be stored here, as shown in Equation 2.16:

$$x(k) = \sum_{n=0}^{n-1} an\varphi n(k) \tag{2.16}$$

where$k$ = 0, 1, 2, …, M−1, $x(k)$: signal, φ_n(k) is the nth element among all N elements, and a_n is the coefficient associated with the nth element.

A number of functions can be used as elements. However, the most commonly used are sine and cosine waveforms, or sinusoids. The Fourier series is the representation of a signal as a sum of sinusoids.

2.6 SINUSOIDS IN EEGS

Sinusoids are defined by three basic elements: amplitude, frequency, and phase angle. For an EEG, the unit of amplitude is most commonly used in μV. The phase angle θ indicates the extent to which the start time of the sinusoids compares to time zero. θ represents the duration to which the sinusoids have shifted relative to the starting point and is expressed as a fraction of the total period. The unit of the phase angle is the °, which is between 0°–360°. Phase angle 360° means that one cycle is fully turned. In reality, the phase angle is expressed in radians. Consider a sinusoid with amplitude A (μV), frequency f (Hz, 1/s), and phase angle θ (rad). Angular velocity or angular frequency $\omega = 2\pi f$ (rad/s).

Then, the time-dependent sine function is given by Equation 2.17:

$$f(t) = A\cdot \sin(\omega\cdot t + \theta) = A\cdot \sin(2\pi\cdot f\cdot t + \theta) \tag{2.17}$$

Here, the unit of time is in seconds (s). The parentheses in the sine function are all in radians; 360° = 2π rad, 180° = π rad, 90° = π/2 rad, and 0° = 0 rad. Figure 2.4 shows a sinusoid with A = 1 μV, f = 1 Hz, θ = 0° (0 rad), and 90° (π/2 rad). Also Figure 2.5 and Figure 2.6 shows sinusoids with varying *A*, *f*, *θ* and their resulting addition respectively.

$$\begin{aligned} x(k) = [&1\cdot \sin(2\pi\cdot 1\cdot k\cdot \Delta_t + 0.5\pi) \\ &+ 1.5\cdot \sin(2\pi\cdot 2\cdot k\cdot \Delta_t + 1.5\pi) \\ &+ 1\cdot \sin(2\pi\cdot 3\cdot k\cdot \Delta_t + 1.7\pi) \\ &+ 2\cdot \sin(2\pi\cdot 4\cdot k\cdot \Delta_t) \\ &+ 1.5\cdot \sin(2\pi\cdot 5\cdot k\cdot \Delta_t + 0.5\pi)] \end{aligned}$$

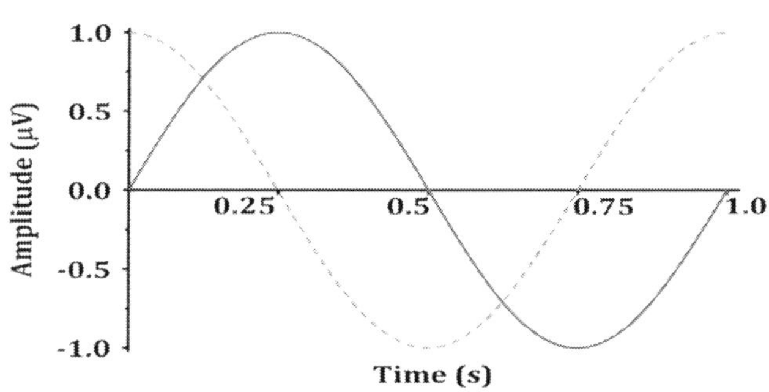

FIGURE 2.4 Sinusoids with amplitude 1, frequency 1, phase angle 0°, and 90° (π/2 rad); f(t) = sin(2π · t): solid line; and sin(2π · t + π/2): dotted line.

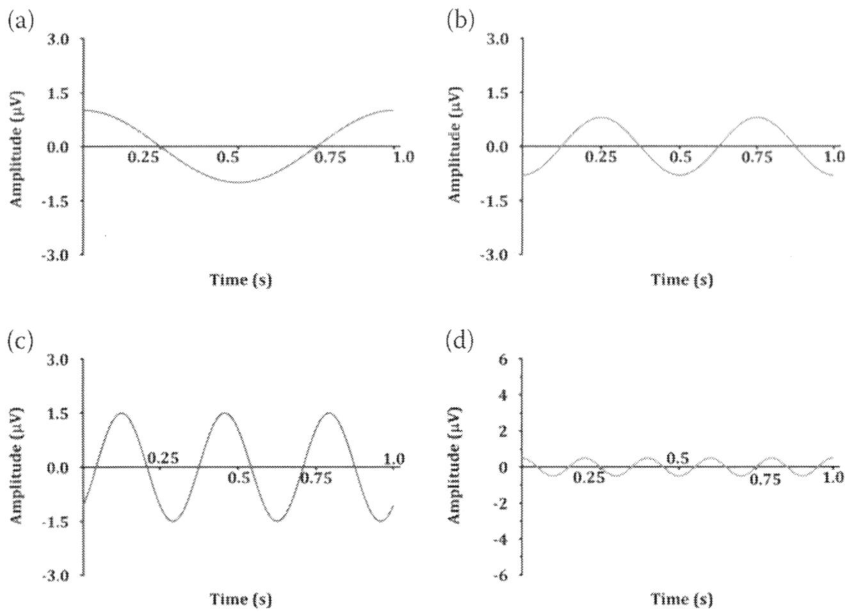

FIGURE 2.5 (a) Sinusoid with frequency 1 Hz, Amplitude 1 and phase angle 90°, (b) Sinusoid with frequency 2 Hz, Amplitude 0.8 and phase angle 270°, (c) Sinusoid with frequency 3 Hz, Amplitude 1.5 and phase angle 315°, (d) Sinusoid with frequency 5 Hz, Amplitude 0.5 and phase angle 90°.

the above summetation of equation can be expressed through Equation 2.18

$$x(k) = \sum_{n=0}^{n=3} An \sin(2\pi{\cdot}fn{\cdot}k{\cdot}\Delta t + \theta n) \tag{2.18}$$

k = 0, 1, 2, 3, …, M−1: represents discrete time of steps $0{\cdot}\Delta_t$, $1{\cdot}\Delta_t$, $2{\cdot}\Delta_t$, …, $(M-1){\cdot}\Delta_t$

n = 0, 1, 2, 3: element

The frequency of the sinusoid of each element is (f_n) = 1, 2, 3, 5 Hz of the sinusoid of each element; the amplitude of the sinusoid of each element is (A_n) = 1, 0.8, 1.5, 0.5 µV; and the phase angle of the sinusoid of each element is (θ_n) = 90° (0.5π rad), 270° (1.5π rad), 315° (1.75π rad), and 90° (0.5π rad).

A generalization of the signal $x(k)$ is the form of the sum of sinusoid elements given by Equation 2.19.

$$x(k) = [1{\cdot} \sin(2\pi{\cdot}1{\cdot}k{\cdot}\Delta_t + 0.5\pi) + 0.8{\cdot} \sin(2\pi{\cdot}2{\cdot}k{\cdot}\Delta_t + 1.5\pi) + 1.5{\cdot} \sin(2\pi{\cdot}3{\cdot}k{\cdot}\Delta_t + 1.75\pi) + 0.5{\cdot} \sin(2\pi{\cdot}5{\cdot}k{\cdot}\Delta_t + 0.5\pi)] \tag{2.19}$$

where k = 0, 1, 2, 3, …, M−1.

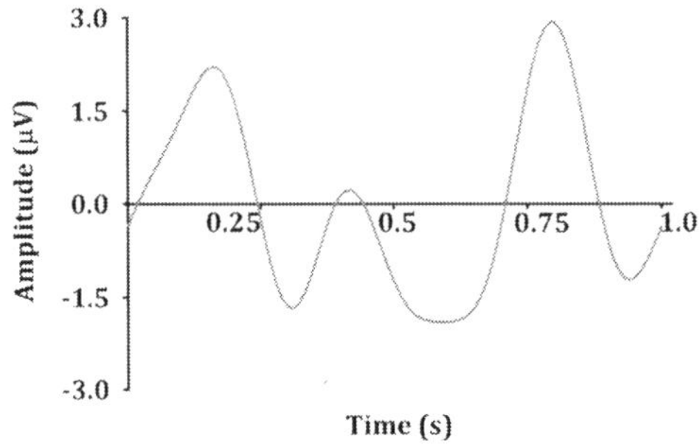

FIGURE 2.6 Addition of the four sinusoids in Figure 2.5 resulted in Figure 2.6.

2.7 FOURIER TRANSFORM AND POWER SPECTRAL ANALYSIS OF EEG SIGNALS

By converting the signal to a Fourier series, each sinusoid element can be studied. This is a common concept in quantitative EEG analysis. EEGs often exhibit delta (δ, 1–4 Hz) theta (θ, 5–8 Hz), alpha (α, 8–13 Hz), and gamma (γ, 30–80 Hz) bands. In general, the conversion of the signal to the amplitude and frequency of the sinusoids of the Fourier series is called the Fourier transform. The Fourier transform converts a time series signal x(t), whose amplitude or power is a function of time, into a frequency series signal X(*f*), whose amplitude or power is a function of frequency. The Fourier transform of the sampled signal x(k) is given by Equation 2.20. The Fourier transform is also a type of integral transform and uses $e^{-ik2\pi f}$ as a kernel function:

$$X(f) = 2M \sum_{k=0}^{m-1} x(k) e^{-ik2\pi f} \tag{2.20}$$

As a result, the Fourier transform X(*f*) consists of a series of discrete values, each corresponding to a particular signal frequency element *f*. The frequency range of X(*f*) is 0 $-f_s/2$ Hz. f_s is the sampling frequency in samples per second. The Fourier transform computed in Equation 2.4 has both positive and negative frequencies, but only positive frequencies are taken for convenience. The frequency resolution of X(*f*) is denoted by f_s/N Hz, where X(*f*) is a few Hz apart, and N is the total number of samples of signal x(k). For example, if x(k) is data for 4 s and f_s = 100 samples/s, N becomes 400, the frequency range of X(*f*) is 0–50 Hz, and the frequency resolution is 0.25 Hz. Therefore, the order of each value of X(*f*) is X(0.00), X(0.25), X(0.50), …, X(50.00). The limitation of the Fourier transformed signal X(*f*) to this frequency range is unavoidable because the sampling rate is not fast enough. To find sinusoids, it is necessary to have at least two sample points within one cycle (reciprocal of the signal frequency, 1/*f*). If at least two sample points cannot be found in one cycle due to slow sampling rate, it appears to be slower than the original analog signal. That is, if the sampling rate is low, a fast analog signal is converted to a slow digital signal. The frequency range should be limited to less than $f_s/2$ to prevent this aliasing error (the high-frequency sinusoids component in the Fourier transform being mistaken for low-frequency sinusoids) while obtaining a signal. If the frequency range is limited to 0 $-f_s/2$ Hz, the Fourier transformed signal X(*f*) will have all the information of the original sampled signal x(k). Therefore, by inverse Fourier transform of X(*f*), the original signal x(k) can be obtained from X(*f*). In other words, when acquiring the signal, the sampling frequency (f_s) should be at least twice the signal frequency (*f*).

The power of each sinusoid element in the Fourier series can be found by calculating the power spectrum *P*(*f*), as given by Equation 2.21:

$$P(f) = |X(f)|^2 \tag{2.21}$$

EEG data can be generally divided into epochs and the power spectrum of the total EEG data is calculated by averaging the power spectrum of all epochs. This reduces the variance of the power spectrum as the frequency resolution becomes low enough to be acceptable. There is only power and frequency information in the power spectrum and no information about the phase angle. The power spectrum can be used to examine how the absolute value and distribution of power changes in response to changes in the central nervous system, and is therefore useful for monitoring and evaluating changes in the central nervous system. For example, in awake normal subjects, most of the power in the EEG is in the alpha and beta bands, but when hypnotic agents are administered, the power distribution shifts to a lower frequency band.

2.8 PHASE COUPLING

Nonlinear systems often have dependent sinusoids in response to sinusoidal input signals. For example, suppose there is a simple nonlinear system where the output γ(k) is the square of the input x(k) as given by Equation 2.22:

$$\gamma(k) = X^2(k) \tag{2.22}$$

If the input signal has sinusoids with frequencies f_1, f_2, respectively, and the phase angles are θ_1, θ_2 (the phase angles are random and independent of each other), Equation 2.23 shows:

$$\text{Input Signal: } x(k) = \cos(2\pi \cdot f_1 \cdot k \cdot \Delta_t + \theta_1) + \cos(2\pi \cdot f_2 \cdot k \cdot \Delta_t + \theta_2) \tag{2.23}$$

Using the formula:

$$(\cos(A) + \cos(B))^2 = 1 + \cos(A + B) + \cos(A - B) + \cos(2A)^2 + \cos(2B)^2$$

The output signal is given in Equation 2.24:

$$\gamma(k) = [1 + \cos[2\pi\cdot(f1 + f2)\cdot k\cdot\Delta t + (\theta 1 + \theta 2)] + \cos[2\pi\cdot(f1 - f2)\cdot k \cdot\Delta t + (\theta 1 - \theta 2)] + 12\cos(2\cdot 2\pi\cdot f1\cdot k\cdot\Delta t + 2\cdot\theta 1) + 12\cos(2\cdot 2\pi\cdot f2\cdot k\cdot\Delta t + 2\cdot\theta 2)] \tag{2.24}$$

Let $\gamma_1(k)$ be the output for the input signal $x_1(k)$ to the system, and $\gamma_2(k)$ be the output for the input signal $x_2(k)$. Here, this system is defined as linear only if the output for the input signal $a\cdot x_1(k) + b\cdot x_2(k)$ *is* $a\cdot\gamma_1(k) + b\cdot\gamma_2(k)$.

One can observe the output signal has components with frequencies of $f_1 + f_2$, $f_1 - f_2$, $2\cdot f_1$, $2\cdot f_2$ in $\gamma(k)$, which are dependent on f_1, f_2 of the input signal. The sinusoids element of the output signal resulting from multiplying the input signal sinusoids element (excluding addition or subtraction) is called the intermodulation product (IMP). The non-multiple output signal sinusoids elements are called fundamental, and there is no such basic form in this example. If a sinusoid element is in the form of an IMP, it is phase-coupled. This process is called quadratic or second-order phase coupling. Phase coupling is a typical feature of nonlinear systems. The ability to analyze the degree of phase coupling within the EEG signal to the external stimulus enables a deeper understanding of the system. For analyzing the central nervous system, correlation analysis between phase coupling of various EEG components can be done. The degree of phase coupling cannot be quantified by power spectral analysis or other quantitative EEG parameters. For example, a signal $\gamma_1(k)$ with the same power spectrum as $\gamma(k)$ of Equation 2.8 can be made by adding frequency $f_1 + f_2, f_1 - f_2$, $2\cdot f_1$, $2\cdot f_2$ to the independent frequency elements, as shown in Equation 2.25:

$$\gamma 1(k) = [1 + \cos(2\pi\cdot fa\cdot k\cdot\Delta t + \theta a) + \cos(2\pi\cdot fb\cdot k\cdot\Delta t + \theta b) + 12\cos(2\pi\cdot fc\cdot k \cdot\Delta t + \theta c) + 12\cos(2\pi\cdot fd\cdot k\cdot\Delta t + \theta d)] \tag{2.25}$$

$$f_a = f_1 + f_2, f_b = f_1 - f_2, f_c = 2\cdot f_1, f_d = 2\cdot f_2$$

θ_a, θ_b, θ_c, θ_d are random and independent.

The signal $\gamma_1(k)$ has a phase structure completely different from that of the phase-correlated signal $\gamma(k)$. However, the power spectrum is the same as the phase-coupled signal. Although these two signals originate from fundamentally different processes, they cannot be distinguished by the power spectrum because the phase information is ignored. Here, all the phase interlocking information is suppressed. The bi-spectral analysis should be used to characterize the degree of phase coupling in the signal.

2.9 PROCESSING OF EEG SIGNALS USING POWER SPECTRAL ANALYSIS

The process of conversion from a raw EEG to a spectrogram is briefly described in Figure 2.7. First, a raw EEG can be separated by sinusoids. This converts the time domain to frequency domain, usually using Fourier transforms. At this time, the unit of the x-axis is the frequency, and the unit of the y-axis is the power. The power of a signal is often expressed as a decibel concept, defined as the amplitude of a given EEG frequency component squared, taken as a log of base 10, and then multiplied by 10, as given in Equation 2.26:

$$\text{Power} = 10 \times \log_{10}(\text{amplitude})^2 \tag{2.26}$$

This can be summarized as follows:

$$\text{Power} = 10 \times \log_{10}(\text{amplitude})^2$$

This is the two-dimensional representation and can be expressed as a three-dimensional spectrogram if considering time (Figure 2.7(d)). This can be expressed in two dimensions, which is called a density spectral array (Figure 2.7(d)). This figure shows at a glance whether the power of a certain frequency increases or decreases with time.

2.10 SUMMARY

In this chapter, we started with the physical modeling of the EEG signal. The Nobel Prize–winning Hodgkin and Huxley's EEG model was discussed along with its mathematical equations. The fundamental concepts and definitions for and understanding of EEG properties and characterizing the signals are related to this model. Further, this chapter discussed the digital signal aspect of the EEG signal, such as digitization of the analog signal to digital signal and fundamental components of the digital EEG signals. Further, the signal was treated partly as stationary and partly non-stationary components. The non-stationary signals can be quantified by measuring some statistics of the signals at different time lags with time. The signals can be deemed stationary if there is no considerable variation in these statistics. Often it is necessary to label the EEG signals into segments of similar characteristics.

The classification of an EEG based on the band of frequency and voltage is particularly meaningful to clinicians and for assessment by neurophysiologists. Within each segment, the signals are considered statistically stationary, usually with similar time and frequency statistics.

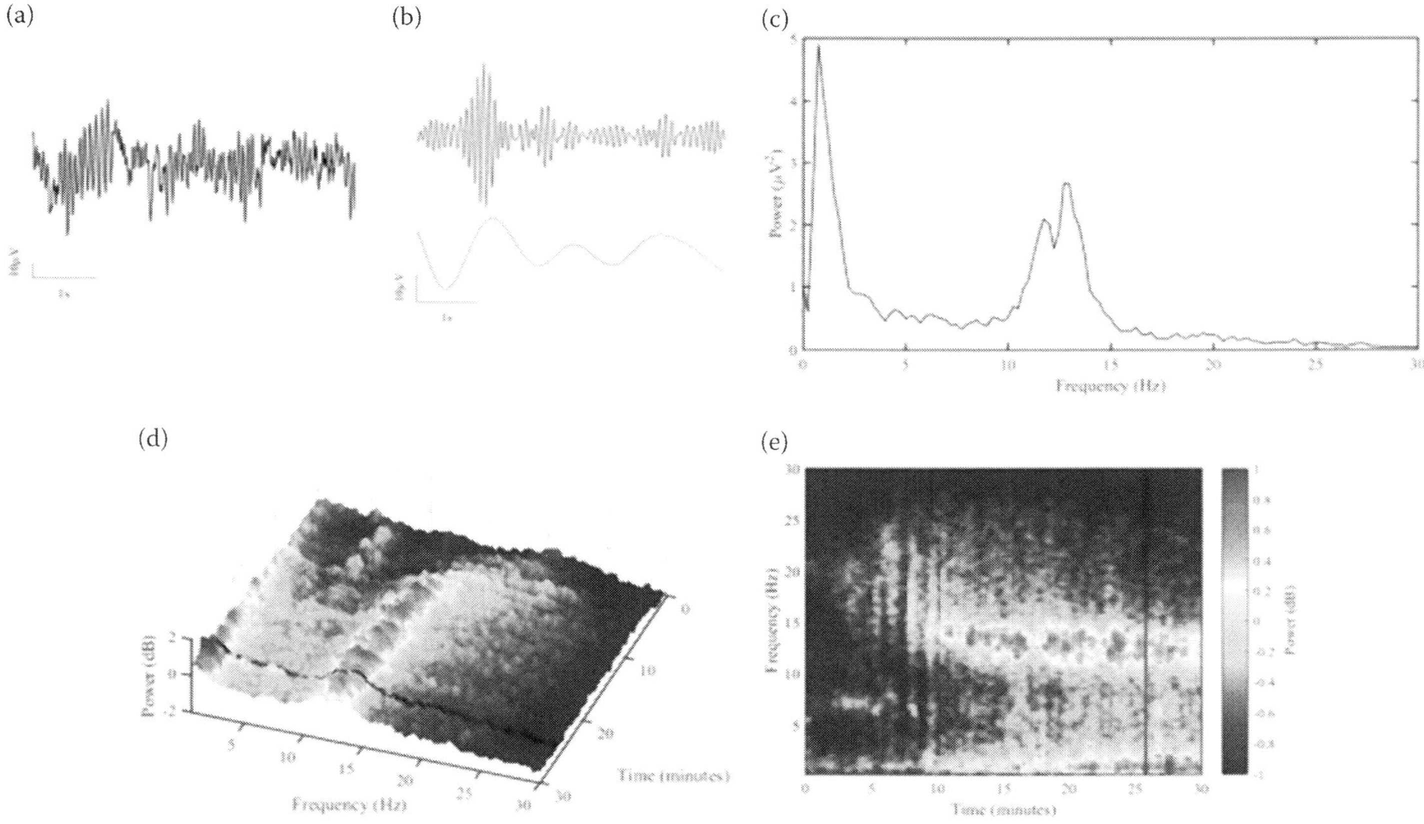

FIGURE 2.7 Analysis process from the raw electroencephalogram (EEG) to the spectrogram. (a) raw EEG, (b) filtered with two major oscillations, (c) power spectral analysis, (d) three-dimensional spectrogram change over 30 minutes, (e) spectrogram change over time presented in two-dimensional space (density spectral array).

The fundamental quantities associated with the EEG signal are its amplitude, frequency, and phase. A study of the properties of these quantities can be performed through analysis of the EEG using various signal processing methods, such as FT and PSD. An EEG signal can be analyzed using many techniques, such as power spectral analysis and Fourier transformation. The physical interpretation of the behavior of these fundamental quantities associated with EEG reveals many different functional properties of the brain.

Exercises

1. What is Hodgkin and Huxley's EEG model? What are the components of the EEG current as per Hodgkin and Huxley's EEG model?
2. Give an analogy of Hodgkin and Huxley's EEG model with that of an ANN (artificial neural network).
3. What are the fundamental characteristics of an EEG signal?
4. How does an analog signal digitized to a digital signal? What is sampling?
5. What are the fundamental attributes of a digital EEG signal?
6. Describe FT. What information does the Fourier transform of a digital signal generate?
7. What is the power spectral density analysis of a signal? What information does a PDA get from an EEG?
8. What is phase coupling? What information about an EEG can be obtained from phase coupling?
9. What is an IMP (inter-modulation product)?

REFERENCES

Forrest, MD 2014 May, 'Can the thermodynamic Hodgkin–Huxley model of voltage-dependent conductance extrapolate for temperature?' (PDF), *Computation*, vol. 2, no. 2, pp. 47–60. doi:10.3390/computation2020047

Hodgkin, AL & Huxley, AF 1952a April, 'The components of membrane conductance in the giant axon of Loligo', *The Journal of Physiology*, vol. 116, no. 4, pp. 473–496.

Hodgkin, AL & Huxley, AF 1952b April, 'Currents carried by sodium and potassium ions through the membrane of the giant axon of Loligo', *The Journal of Physiology*, vol. 116, no. 4, pp. 449–472.

Hodgkin, AL & Huxley, AF 1952c April, 'The dual effect of membrane potential on sodium conductance in the giant axon of Loligo', *The Journal of Physiology*, vol. 116, no. 4, pp. 497–506.

Hodgkin, AL & Huxley, AF 1952d August, 'A quantitative description of membrane current and its application to conduction and excitation in nerve', *The Journal of Physiology*, vol. 117, no. 4, pp. 500–544. doi:10.1113/jphysiol.1952.sp004764. PMC 1392413. PMID 12991237.

Hodgkin, AL, Huxley, AF & Katz, B 1952 April, 'Measurement of current-voltage relations in the membrane of the giant axon of Loligo', *The Journal of Physiology*, vol. 116, no. 4, pp. 424–448.

3 Signal Processing for EEGs

This chapter discusses the prominent signal pre-processing and processing techniques used for EEG signal processing. Also discussed are some of the feature extraction techniques and feature classification techniques, which are the end objectives of different applications such as medical diagnostics, brain computer interface (BCI), Internet of Things (IoT), and Internet of Medical Things (IoMT), etc.

The mathematical aspects of each of the processing and transformation are discussed to make the reader understand how the signal is transformed to obtain the physical characteristic such as the voltage, amplitude, frequency, and the power spectra of the EEG signal.

3.1 INTRODUCTION

EEG signals are a measure of the electrical activity of the brain recorded in space and time. The cortical nerve cell inhibitory and excitatory postsynaptic potentials generate the EEG signals. These postsynaptic potentials summate in the cortex and extend to the scalp surface where they are recorded as an EEG. A typical EEG signal, measured from the scalp, will have an amplitude of about 10 μV to 100 μV and a frequency in the range of 1 Hz to about 100 Hz. While recording the signal, it encounters a number of interferences and/or artifacts that get added as noise, such as eye blinks and power line interferences to name a few. Thus, EEG signals are highly non-Gaussian, non-stationary, and have a nonlinear nature (Subha et al 2010). The brain signals are highly complex and random in nature. Their characteristics strongly depend on the age and mental state of the subject. The occurrence of symptoms is also random on a time scale. Hence, understanding the behavior and dynamics of billions of interconnected neurons involves several linear and nonlinear signal processing techniques and their correlation to the physiological events.

The pre-processing techniques, if implemented correctly, will help us give better information about the activity in the brain and also enable us to use it to control/detect/remove certain points of interest e.g., blink artifact removal.

A block diagram describing EEG signal processing, which depicts the sections of this review, is shown in Figure 3.1.

DOI: 10.1201/9781003241386-3

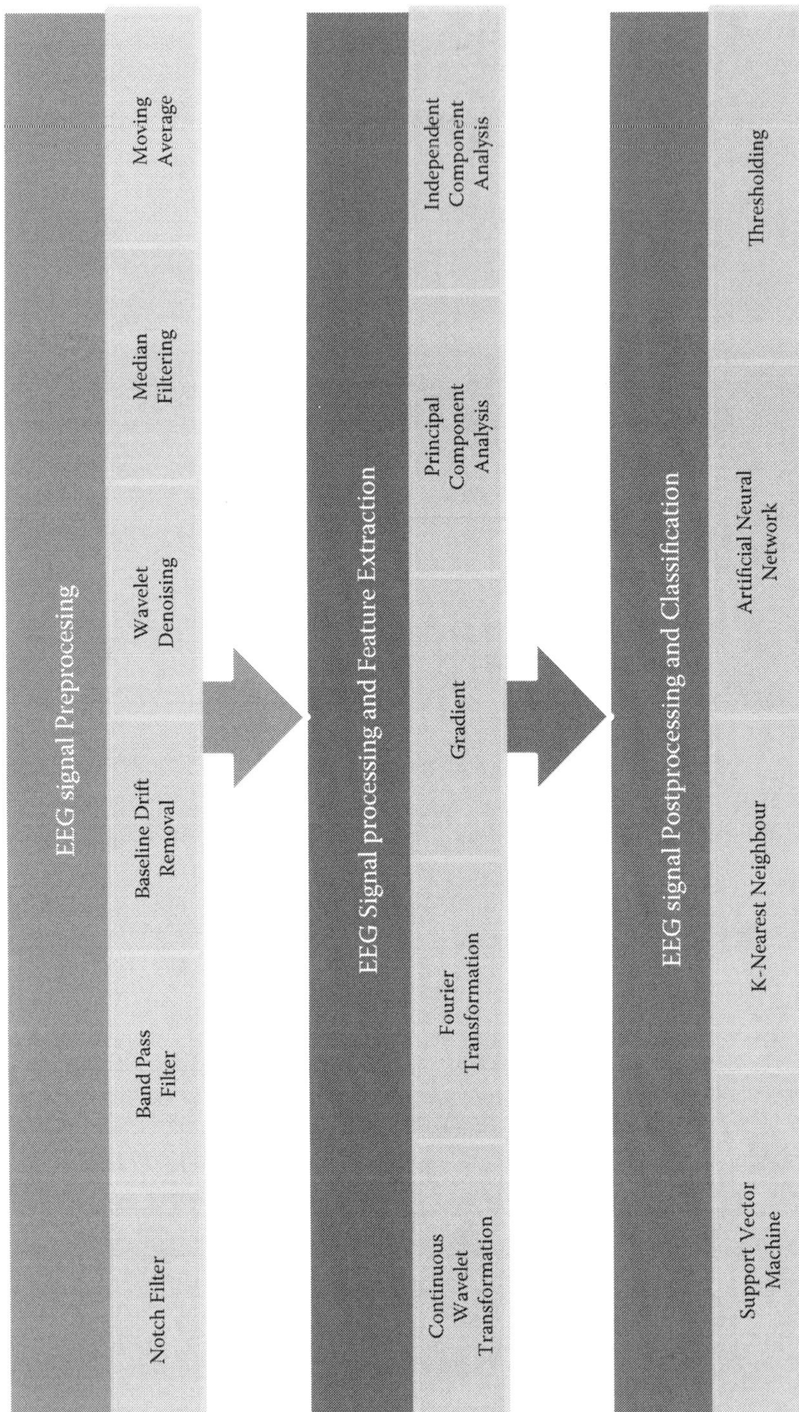

FIGURE 3.1 Block diagram for EEG signal processing techniques.

The processing of EEG can be segregated into three different phases: pre-processing, processing, and post-processing. Various signal processing techniques generally used in these phases are surveyed and gathered from different research literature available.

3.2 FILTERS FOR PROCESSING EEG SIGNALS

Processing of the EEG signal involves a careful analysis of the signal and differs depending on the application or the type of information required for its interpretation. Following are a few of the processing techniques that are commonly used to extract useful information or remove the unwanted noise from it.

3.2.1 Band-Pass Filtering

The most ideal filter design would be one that removes all of the electrical noise or artifact from the EEG and only allows true cerebral activity to pass through. Unfortunately, no such "smart" filter exists; filters can only remove waves according to rigid mathematical rules. Luckily, there are good rationales for filtering out certain components of EEG signals using fairly simple mathematical assumptions. These assumptions are based on the idea that the brain only generates EEG waves within a certain range of frequencies and that any activity outside that range (unusually slow activity and unusually fast activity) is not likely to have originated from the activity of the cerebral origin. Indeed, one of the general assumptions of EEG filter designs is that activities well below 1 Hz and well above 35 Hz do not arise from the brain and likely represent electrical noise or artifact.

EEG filters are typically set up so that one filter rejects the majority of very high-frequency activity and another filter rejects the majority of very low-frequency activity. The range of frequencies between these unwanted high and low frequencies that is allowed to pass through the filter setup is referred to as the band-pass. Figure 3.2 describes the frequency characteristics of the band-pass filter.

3.2.2 Notch Filter

Notch filters are certain filters that can stop signals of a certain frequency to be filtered out. After recording raw EEG signal, one of the most apparent noises that will be present in the signal is the power line signal frequency. A notch filter at 60 Hz/50 Hz is used to filter out power line noise with minimal disruption to the rest of the signal. As explained in the Figure 3.3, f_c (characteristic frequency) should be 60 Hz.

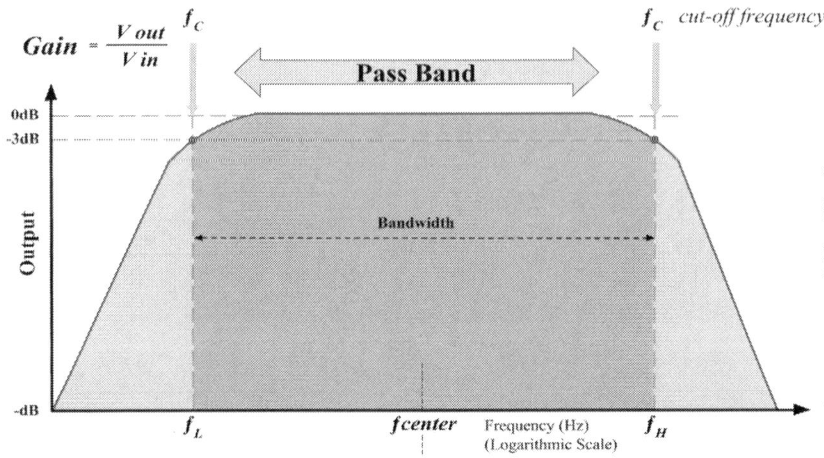

FIGURE 3.2 Frequency characteristics of band-pass filter.

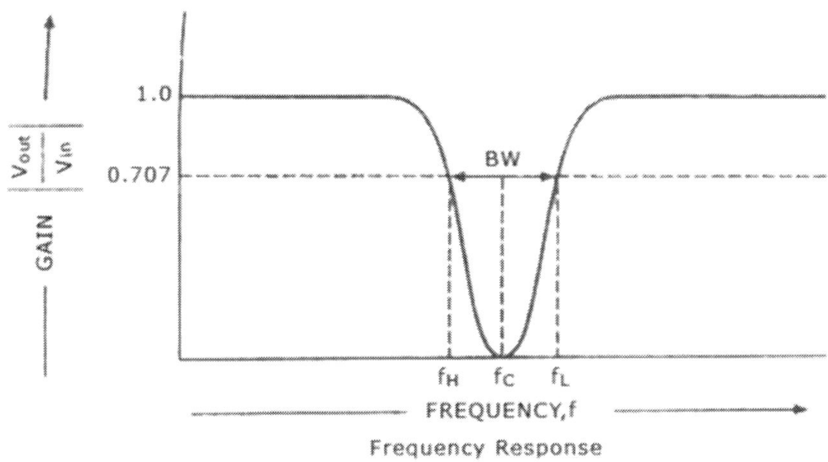

FIGURE 3.3 Notch filter frequency response.

3.2.3 Continuous Wavelet Transform (CWT)

A wavelet is a wave-like oscillation with an amplitude that starts out at zero, increases, and then decreases back to zero. Unlike the sines used in a Fourier transform for decomposition of a signal, wavelets are generally much more concentrated in time. They usually provide an analysis of the signal, which is localized in both time and frequency, whereas a Fourier transform is localized only in frequency. Examples for wavelets are given in Figure 3.4.

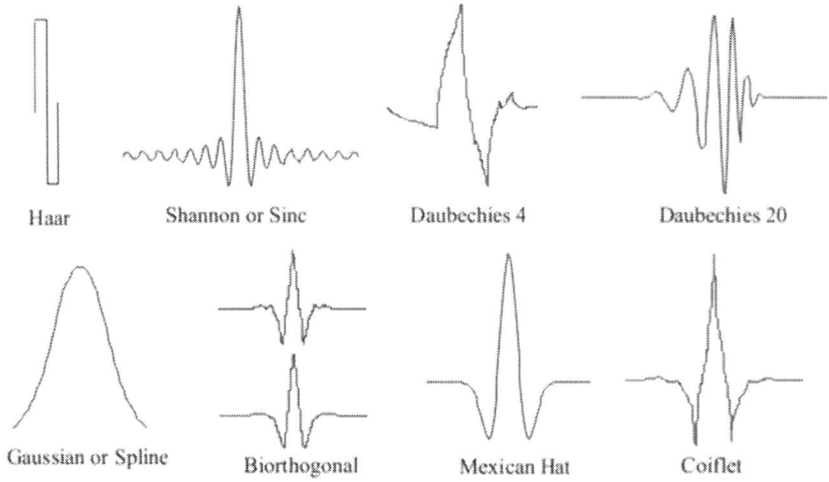

FIGURE 3.4 Different wavelets used for a wavelet transform.

The original signal is transformed using predefined wavelets in a wavelet transform. The wavelet transform is classified into a discrete wavelet transform and a continuous wavelet transform.

Given a mother wavelet ψ(t) (which can be considered simply as a basis function of L2), the continuous wavelet transform (CWT) of a function x(t) (assuming that $x^2 \in$ L2) is defined as (Equation 3.1):

$$X(a, b) = \frac{1}{\sqrt{a}} \int_{-\infty}^{\infty} \psi\left(\frac{t-b}{a}\right) x(t)dt \tag{3.1}$$

3.2.3.1 Mallat's Algorithm

In the case of DWT, assuming that the length of the signal satisfies N = 2J for some positive J, the transform can be computed efficiently, using Mallat's algorithm (Moghim & Corne 2014), which has a complexity of O(N). Essentially the algorithm is a fast hierarchical scheme for deriving the required inner products (which appear in [3.1], as a function of a and b) using a set of consecutive low- and high-pass filters, followed by a decimation. This results in a decomposition of the signal into different scales that can be considered different frequency bands. The low-pass (LP) and high-pass (HP) filters used in this algorithm are determined according to the mother wavelet in use. The outputs of the LP filters are referred to as approximation coefficients and the outputs of the

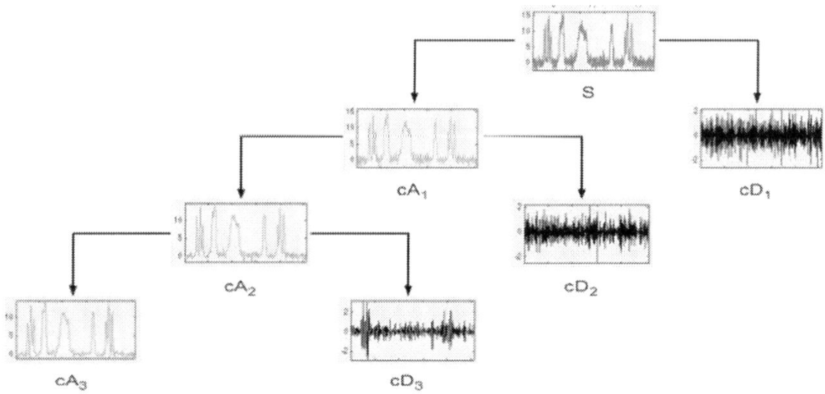

FIGURE 3.5 Wavelet decomposition at level 3.

HP filters are referred to as detail coefficients. A demonstration of the process of three-level decomposition of a signal can be seen in Figure 3.5.

There are many types of wavelets. Daubechies wavelet is described by a maximal number of vanishing moments for some given support. A Haar wavelet is an order of rescaled square-shaped function that together form a wavelet family. Symlet wavelets are an improved version of Daubechies wavelets with increased symmetry. Coiflets wavelets have scaling functions with vanishing moments. Signal reconstruction means reconstructing the original sequence from the thresholded wavelet detail coefficients that leads to a denoised version of the original signal. Inverse discrete wavelet transform (IDWT) is used to reconstruct the original signal. Therefore, wavelet transform is a reliable and better technique than the Fourier transform technique.

3.2.3.2 Wavelet Families

- **Daubachies**: Daubechies family wavelets are signed dbN (N is the order). This wavelet belongs to orthogonal wavelets.
- **Coiflets**: Discrete wavelets designed by Ingrid Daubechies to have a scaling function with vanishing moments. The scaling function and the wavelet function must be normalized by a common factor.
- **Symlet**: The symlet family wavelets are signed symN (N is the order). The symlets are nearly symmetrical, orthogonal, and bi-orthogonal wavelets suggested by Daubechies as modifications to the db family. The properties of the two wavelet families are similar.
- **Biorthogonal: Biorthogonal** filters state a superset of orthogonal wavelet filters. The bi-orthogonal family wavelets are signed as bior. Bi-orthogonal wavelet transform has frequently been used in numerous image processing applications because it makes possible multi-resolution analysis and does not produce redundant information.

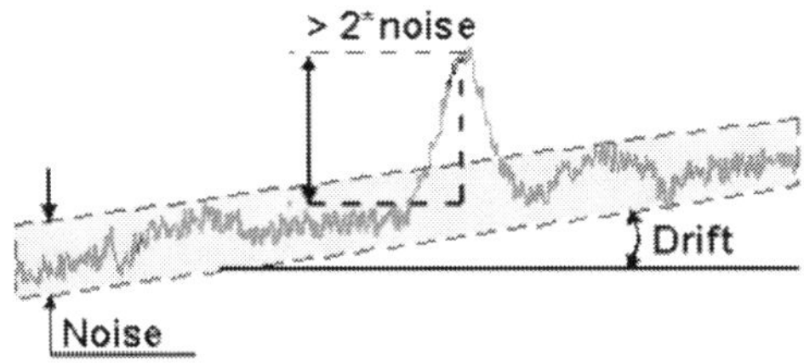

FIGURE 3.6 Baseline drift.

3.2.4 Baseline Drift Removal

Baseline correction belongs to one of the standard procedures in ERP research (Alday 2019). The sources of baseline wander may be different, but it always appears as a low-frequency artifact that introduces slow oscillations in the recorded signal. Baseline is due to brain activity, muscle tension, sweating, eye and head movements, electrode movement (in the case of EEGs), or other noise sources (Fasano & Villani 2014) (Figure 3.6).

Although baseline noise may be reduced by properly preparing skin and using suitable electrodes and an electrode–gel combination, a pre-processing step for its removal is still required. In an EOG, de-trending is achieved using a technique devised for ECG signals, which is based on wavelet decomposition. As observed in Figure 3.6 the baseline is seen to drift up due to the increase in the DC offset value. The change in the DC offset that makes a gradual rise/fall of the signal is known as baseline drift.

3.2.5 Wavelet Denoising

Wavelets localize features in your data to different scales; you can preserve important signals or image features while removing noise. The basic idea behind wavelet denoising, or wavelet thresholding, is that the wavelet transform leads to a sparse representation for many real-world signals and images. What this means is that the wavelet transform concentrates signal and image features in a few large-magnitude wavelet coefficients. Wavelet coefficients that are small in value are typically noise and you can "shrink" those coefficients or remove them without affecting the signal or image quality. After you threshold the coefficients, you reconstruct the data using the inverse wavelet transform.

The most general model for the noisy signal has the following form (Equation 3.2):

$$s(n) = f(n) + \sigma e(n) \tag{3.2}$$

where time n is equally spaced. In the simplest model, suppose that $e(n)$ is a Gaussian white noise $N(0,1)$, and the noise level σ is equal to 1. The denoising objective is to suppress the noise part of the signal s and to recover f.

The denoising procedure has three steps:

1. **Decomposition:** Choose a wavelet, and choose a level N. Compute the wavelet decomposition of the signal *s* at level N.
2. **Detail coefficients thresholding:** For each level from 1 to N, select a threshold and apply soft thresholding to the detail coefficients.
3. **Reconstruction:** Compute wavelet reconstruction based on the original approximation coefficients of level N and the modified detail coefficients of levels from 1 to N.

3.2.6 Median Filtering

Median filtering (Paranjape 2009) is a common nonlinear method for noise suppression that has unique characteristics. It does not use convolution to process the image with a kernel of coefficients. Rather, in each position of the kernel frame, a pixel of the input image contained in the frame is selected to become the output pixel located at the coordinates of the kernel center. The kernel frame is centered on each pixel (m, n) of the original image, and the median value of pixels within the kernel frame is computed. The pixel at the coordinates (m, n) of the output image is set to this median value. In general, median filters do not have the same smoothing characteristics as the mean filter (Gonzalez & Wintz 1987). Features that are smaller than half the size of the median filter kernel are completely removed by the filter. Large discontinuities such as edges and large changes in image intensity are not affected in terms of gray-level intensity by the median filter, although their positions may be shifted by a few pixels. This nonlinear operation of the median filter allows significant reduction of specific types of noise. For example, "pepper-and-salt noise" may be removed completely from an image without attenuation of significant edges or image characteristics. Figure 3.7 presents typical results of median filtering.

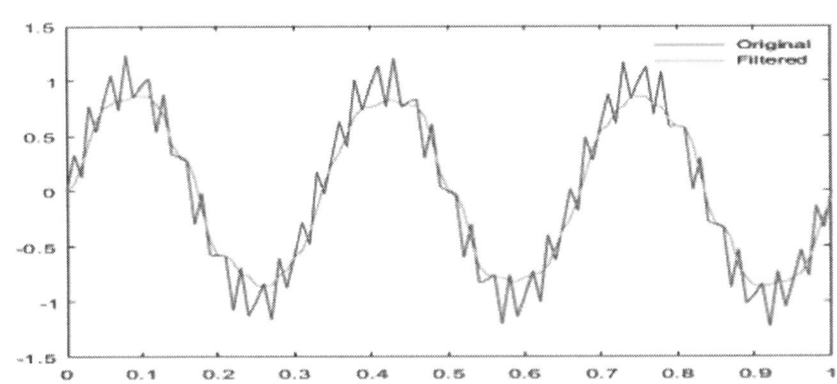

FIGURE 3.7 Comparison between median-filtered signal and the original signal.

3.2.7 Moving Average

In statistics, a moving average (rolling average or running average) is a calculation to analyze data points by creating a series of averages of different subsets of the full data set. It is also called a moving mean (MM) or rolling mean and is a type of finite impulse response filter. Variations include simple and cumulative, or weighted, forms.

Given a series of numbers and a fixed subset size, the first element of the moving average is obtained by taking the average of the initial fixed subset of the number series. Then the subset is modified by "shifting forward"; that is, excluding the first number of the series and including the next value in the subset.

A moving average is commonly used with time series data to smooth out short-term fluctuations and highlight longer-term trends or cycles. The threshold between short-term and long-term depends on the application, and the parameters of the moving average will be set accordingly. For example, it is often used in technical analysis of financial data, like stock prices, returns, or trading volumes. It is also used in economics to examine gross domestic product, employment, or other macroeconomic time series. Mathematically, a moving average is a type of convolution and so it can be viewed as an example of a low-pass filter used in signal processing. When used with non-time series data, a moving average filters higher-frequency components without any specific connection to time, although typically some kind of ordering is implied. Viewed simplistically, it can be regarded as smoothing the data. Figure 3.8 demonstrates the comparison of the two processes.

3.3 TRANSFORMATION METHODS USED IN EEG SIGNAL PROCESSING

In the nonparametric approach of extraction of features from EEG signals, both a global Fourier transform (FT) and wavelet transformation can be used for the spectral analysis. The biofeatures extracted from each of these transformations are very useful in discriminating the EEG signal between epileptic and normal. Generally the FT gives an average spectral plot over the time period considered. On the other hand, wavelets are mathematical functions that divide the data into different frequency components and then analyze each component with a resolution matched to their scale. Thus, instead of working on a single time or frequency scale, they work on a multi-scale basis (Konstantinidis et al 2015). Wavelets offer a trade-off between time and frequency resolution and they are superior to traditional fast Fourier transform (FFT) methods when it comes to analyzing data that contains discontinuities and sharp spikes. In addition, the time-windowed version of the wavelets offer a scheme that allows for further refinement of the method in cases where time-locked events might be important. When wavelets were compared to the STFT technique (Konstantinidis et al 2015), the results showed that the STFT is computationally faster but wavelets give more accurate results, especially in the detection of epileptic seizures and in

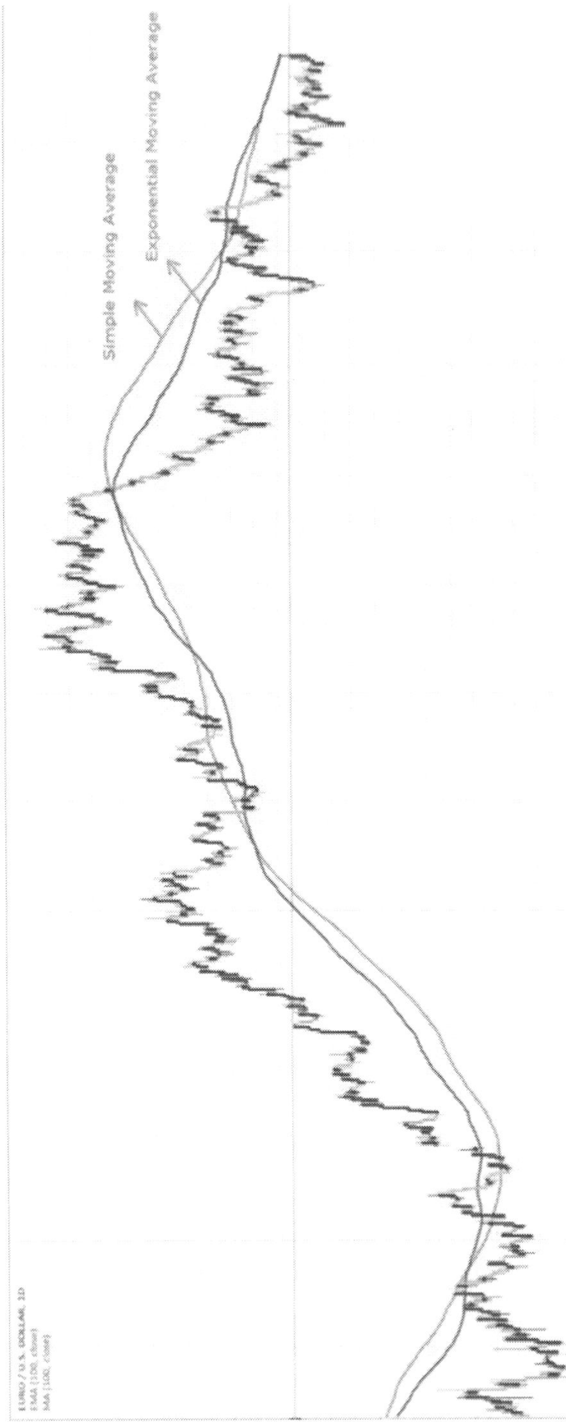

FIGURE 3.8 Simple moving average vs exponential moving average vs original signal.

EEG signal classification. For these reasons, the wavelets are opted for analysis of EEG in addition to the application of a global FT to extract power spectral features within predefined frequency bands like that of EEG signals. Therefore, a wavelet is used for the presence of the particular EEG rhythms in the EEG signal, which are then used for classification purposes.

3.3.1 Fourier Transformation

The FT transforms an EEG signal in the time domain into its frequency domain representation. By definition, a signal has a discrete Fourier transform. The power spectral density for such a signal is then estimated . This spectrum is then used to extract biomarkers, which are then fed to a classifier to distinguish between the two populations. Biomarkers are found by calculating the total energy for each of six predefined frequency bands: delta (0–4 Hz), theta (4–8 Hz), alpha (8–13 Hz), beta (13–30 Hz), gamma1 (30–45 Hz), and gamma2 (45–90 Hz), where the biomarker is at the frequency band and is the sampling frequency.

3.3.2 Wavelet Transform (WT)

Over the past decade, the WT has been developed into an important tool for analysis of time series data that contains non-stationary power at many different frequencies, such as the EEG signal, seismic data, and other biosignals. WT has proven to be a powerful feature extraction method for EEG signals because of the frequency range, such as delta (0–4 Hz), theta (4–8 Hz), alpha (8–13 Hz), beta (13–30 Hz), gamma1 (30–45 Hz), and gamma2 (45–90 Hz). In particular, WT is very useful in isolating and observing the epileptic signal characteristic during seizure development and can describe it in terms of the relative wavelet energies. The WT is more suitable for analyzing transient signals because both frequency (scales) and time information can be obtained in good resolution.

The continuous wavelet transform (CWT) was preferred in analyzing EEG signals, so that the time and scale parameters can be considered as continuous variables. In the CWT, the notion of scale is introduced as an alternative to frequency, leading to the so-called time-scale representation. The CWT of a discrete sequence is given by Equation 3.1.

3.3.3 Discrete Cosine Transformation (DCT)

DCT is a transformation method for converting a time series signal into basic frequency components. Low-frequency components are concentrated in first coefficients, while high-frequency components are in the last ones. The DCT input X(t) is a set of N data values (EEG samples, audio samples, or other data) and the output Y(u) is a set of N discrete cosine transform coefficients. The one-dimensional DCT for a list of N real numbers is expressed by Equation 3.3:

$$Y(u) = \sqrt{\frac{2}{N}} \propto (u) \sum_{t=o}^{N-1} x(t)\left(\mathrm{Cos}\left(\frac{\pi(2t+1).\, u}{2N}\right)\right) \tag{3.3}$$

$$\text{where} \propto (u) = \begin{cases} \frac{1}{\sqrt{2}}, & U = 0 \\ 1, & U > 0 \end{cases}$$

The coefficient Y(u) is called the DC coefficient and the rest are referred to as AC coefficients (AL-Quraishi et al 2018). The DC coefficient contains a mean value of the original signal. Inverse DCT takes transform coefficients Y(u) as input and converts them back into time series f(x). For a list of N DCT coefficients, an inverse transform is expressed by the following formula (Equation 3.4):

$$X(t) = \sqrt{\frac{2}{N}} \propto (u) \sum_{u=o}^{N-1} Y(u)\left(\mathrm{Cos}\left(\frac{\pi(2x+1).\, u}{2N}\right)\right) \tag{3.4}$$

In this formula, notations are the same as in Equation 3.3. DCT exhibits good energy compaction for correlated signals. If the input data consists of correlated quantities, most of the N transform coefficients produced by the DCT are zeros or small numbers, and only a few coefficients are large. These small numbers can be quantized coarsely, usually down to zero. Since an EEG has low-frequency oscillations, most of the relevant information is compressed into the first coefficients, while the last ones usually contain noise.

During the implementation of the transform, small values of N, such as 3, 4, or 6, result in many small sets of data items and small sets of coefficients where the energy of the original signal is concentrated in a few coefficients, but there are not enough small coefficients to quantize. Large values of N result in a few large sets of data. The problem in this case is that individual data items of a large set are normally not correlated and therefore result in a set of transform coefficients where all the coefficients are large. Most data compression methods that employ the DCT use the value of N = 8.

3.3.4 Continuous Wavelet Transformation (CWT)

The question "Can wavelet transform be used for feature extraction from EEG signal?" has been answered positively through many experiments and reported by many research literature. In this section, we discuss the usefulness of wavelet transform as a feature extraction method from EEG signal for both seizure patients and non-seizure patients. Experiments have suggested that wavelet transform in combination with non-negative matrix factorization methods have promising result for feature extraction of EEG signal.

Human body movements can be reflected in brain signals and collected noninvasively with electroencephalography (EEG). Motor-related signals include sensory motor rhythms (also known as the Mu wave) in the upper-alpha band of 8–13 Hz and slow cortical potentials (SCPs) in the low frequency range of 0.1–5 Hz. This study compares the two signals for decoding finger movements. Human subjects were asked to individually lift each of the five digits of their right hand, at the rate of one every 10 s. EEG was recorded using a bipolar montage between ipsilateral and contralateral motorcortices. Electromyograms were obtained for identifying movement onsets. Linear discriminant analysis (LDA) generated significant performance with SCPs but not with Mu. Meanwhile, continuous wavelet transform (CWT) was applied to SCPs or Mu to create a spectrogram for each finger, showing distinctive amplitude and phase patterns. A dprime-based weighting algorithm was used to extract time-frequency features. With a template-matching paradigm, both SCP and Mu spectrograms yielded significant classification accuracies for multiple subjects, with the highest being >50% (chance = 20%). Interestingly, the index finger was better distinguished with Mu for most of the subjects, whereas the ring finger was better distinguished with SCPs. The CWT algorithm outperformed LDA by better decoding the thumb. This study suggests that the time-frequency characteristics of a single-channel EEG, when phase is preserved, contain critical information on finger movements. SCPs and Mu seem to work in an independent but complementary manner.

3.3.5 Discrete Wavelet Transformation (DWT)

In this section, we discuss the usefulness of DWT to transform and analyze the EEG signal is discussed. The coefficients derived from EEG signal using DWT as features for emotion recognition from EEG signals is highly applied in different applications. Other feature extraction methods used power spectra density values derived from Fourier transform or sub-band energy and entropy derived from Wavelet Transform for analysis of EEG. These feature extraction methods eliminate temporal information present in the signal, which are essential for analyzing EEG signals. The DWT coefficients obtained from EEG represent the degree of correlation between the analyzed signal and the wavelet function at different instances of time; therefore, DWT coefficients contain temporal information of the analyzed signal. The feature extracted from EEG using DWT method fully utilizes the simultaneous time-frequency analysis by preserving the temporal information in the DWT coefficients. Therefore coefficient obtained from DWT applied on EEG is highly useful for emotion recognition of the subject. In an experiment the input EEG signals obtained from two electrodes according to 10–20 system: F(p1) and F(p2). Visual stimuli from International Affective Picture System (IAPS) were used to induce two emotions: happy and sad. Two classifiers were used: extreme learning machine (ELM) and support vector machine (SVM). Experimental results confirmed that the DWT coefficients obtained from the EEG signal captured in the experiment showed improved performance in detecting emotion of the subject compared to other features and methods.

3.4 FEATURE EXTRACTION

There are different feature extraction techniques used (Al-Fahoum & Al-Fraihat 2014) for extracting significant features from the transformed EEG signal. Some of the prominent techniques discussed in this section are (a) principal component analysis (b) independent component analysis and (c) Hjorth parameters.

3.4.1 Principal Component Analysis (PCA)

Principal component analysis (PCA) is the most widely used method for pattern recognition and feature extraction. It is used as the variable reduction procedure. PCA is used when there are a large number of variables and some redundancy occurs in the variables. Redundancy means that some of the variables are correlated with one another. Due to this redundancy, it is possible to reduce the observed variables into a smaller number of principal components that will account for most of the variance in the observed variables. A principal component can be defined as a linear combination of optimally weighted observed variables. PCA is used for analyzing data and finding the patterns. It is a dominant tool for data compression and it projects higher-dimensional data to lower-dimensional data.

3.4.2 Independent Component Analysis (ICA)

The blind source separation has been widely used in many practical areas of modern signal processing. Based on the blind source separation, the independent source signals can be recovered after the signals are linearly mixed with an unknown medium and recorded at N sensors. The concept of independent component analysis (ICA) was described as maximizing the degree of statistical independence among outputs using contrast functions approximated with the Edge worth expansion of the Kullback-Leibler divergence. This is in contrast with de-correlation techniques such as PCA, which ensure that the output pairs are uncorrelated. ICA imposes the much stronger criterion that the multivariate probability density function of output variables factorizes. To find such a factorization, it is required that the mutual information between all variable pairs becomes zero. The de-correlation only takes account of second-order statistics, but the mutual information depends on all higher-order cumulants of the output variables (Sun et al 2005).

To deal with the problem of EEG signal preprocessing, artifact cancellation, and source localization, it is always difficult due to the fact that the determination of a brain electrical source from patterns collected from the scalp is mathematically underdetermined. Recent efforts to identify EEG sources have focused mostly on performing spatial segregation and localization of source activity. Using the ICA algorithm, the problem of both source identification and source localization have been investigated. The ICA algorithm derives independent sources from highly correlated EEG signals statistically and does not regard the physical location or configuration of the source generators of EEG signals.

3.4.3 Hjorth Parameters

Hjorth parameters of EEG signals describe the general characteristics of an EEG trace in a few quantitative terms. Its descriptive parameters are entirely based on time, but they can be derived also from the statistical moments of the power spectrum. Thus, the method provides a bridge between a physical time domain interpretation and the conventional frequency domain description. Further, the parameters are based on the concept of variance, giving them an additive property so that the measured values pertain also to any basic elements from which a complex curve may be composed by superposition.

Hjorth parameters are indicators of statistical properties used in signal processing in the time domain introduced by Bo Hjorth (1970). The parameters are activity, mobility, and complexity. They are commonly used in the analysis of electroencephalography signals for feature extraction.

a. **Hjorth Activity:** The activity parameter represents the signal power, the variance of a time function. This can indicate the surface of a power spectrum in the frequency domain given by Equation 3.5:

$$\text{Activity} = \text{Var}(\text{x}[\text{t}]) \tag{3.5}$$

where x[t] is the EEG signal.

b. **Hjorth Mobility:** The mobility parameter represents the mean frequency or the proportion of standard deviation of the power spectrum. This is defined as the square root of variance of the first derivative of the signal X[t] divided by variance of the signal x[t] given by Equation 3.6:

$$Mobility = \sqrt{\frac{Var\left(\frac{\partial x(t)}{\partial t}\right)}{Var(x[t\})}} \tag{3.6}$$

c. **Hjorth Complexity:** Similarly, the Hjorth complexity parameter represents the change in frequency (Equation 3.7). The parameter compares the signal's similarity to a pure sine wave, where the value converges to 1 if the signal is more similar.

$$Complexity = \frac{Mobility\left(\frac{\partial x(t)}{\partial t}\right)}{Mobility(x[t\})} \tag{3.7}$$

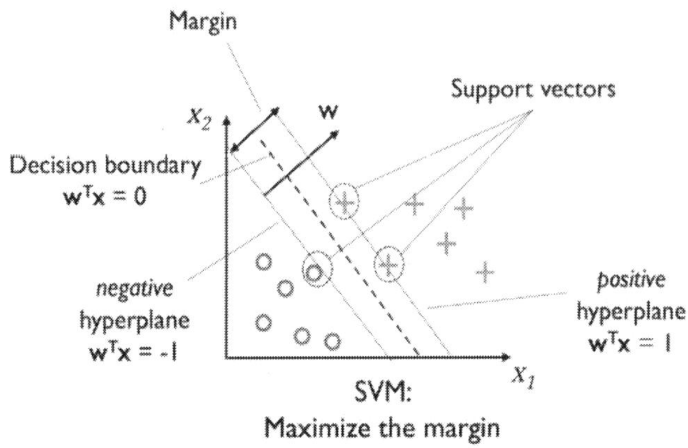

FIGURE 3.9 Illustration of trained hyperplane.

3.5 EEG SIGNAL CLASSIFICATION TECHNIQUES

Classifying the EEG signal into its characteristic features or signal type helps in interpretation of the state of the human mind. Also the classified signal are used for interpretation in the state of the subject and are mapped to different intended commands in driving different devices.Therefore, quick and accurate classification of EEG signal is an important prerequisite towards driving IoT, IoMT and BCI. In this section three techniques viz. SVM, KNN and ANN often used in EEG signal classificationare discussed.

3.5.1 Support Vector Machines (SVMs)

A support vector machine (Figure 3.9) is a machine learning model used for classification and regression analysis. When a SVM is used for classification, it separates a given set of binary labeled training data and a hyperplane that is maximally distance from them. Assume the input data is $x^j = (x^{1j} \ldots x^{nj})$ by the realization of the random vector x^j while φ is the map mapping the feature space to a label space y, where label space contains many vectors, mathematically labeled as $\{(x^1, y^1), \ldots (x^m, y^m)\}$. The SVM learning algorithm finds a hyperplane (w, b) such that the quantity:

$$\gamma = min_t y^i \{<\mathbf{w}, \phi(\mathbf{x}^i) > -b\} \tag{3.8}$$

is maximized. In Equation 3.8, the dimension of φ is the same as the dimension of the label y and $< w, f(x^i) > -b$ corresponds to the distance between point x^i and the decision boundary. γ is the margin and b is a real number. The kernel of this function is $Ki, j = < \varphi(x^i), \varphi(x^j) >$. Given a new data x to classify, a label is assigned according to its relationship to the decision boundary, and the corresponding decision function is expressed as the following (Equation 3.9):

$$f(x) = \text{sign}(<w, \varphi(x)> -b) \tag{3.9}$$

3.5.2 K-Nearest Neighbor (KNN)

K-NN classification is a non-parametric model that is described as instance-based learning, in which the model is characterized by memorizing the training data set (Isa et al 2017). KNN is also a typical example of a lazy learner. It is called lazy not because of its apparent simplicity, but because it does not learn a discriminative function from the training data but memorized the training data set instead. Lazy learning is a special case of instance-based learning that is associated with zero cost during the learning process. The K-NN algorithm is suitable to classify EEG data as it is a robust technique for large, noisy data. The sample is the data classified by the majority vote of its neighbor's class. In order to determine the class, this algorithm requires training data and a predefined k value as it will search through the training sample space for the k-most similar samples based on a similarity measure of a distance function. The value of k and distance metric will affect the result of classification. Figure 3.10 illustrates the concept of a K-NN algorithm when applied to the distance metric to determine the appropriate class of new data with k = 9. The data to be classified is at point (0.6, 0.45), which is shown with "X." The big circle with dotted line represents the distance metric using Euclidean distance computation. It has two possible classes: circle class with six instances and triangle class with three instances. The algorithm will classify mark "X" to the circle class as the circle class has the majority of data within the radius.

3.5.3 Artificial Neural Network (ANN)

Artificial neural network (ANN) is a paradigm that is related to biological networks and tries to mimic the structure of the human brain (Lekshmi et al 2014).

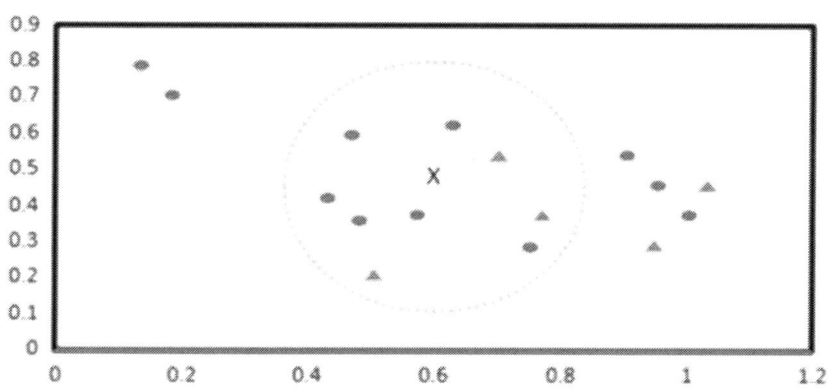

FIGURE 3.10 KNN applied with k = 9.

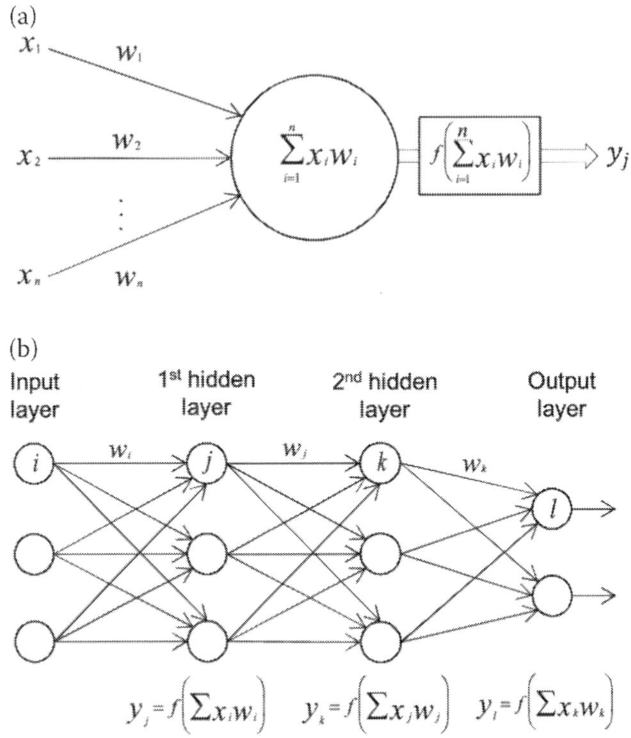

FIGURE 3.11 (a) Operation of one neural unit of the neural network. Here, "f" is a predefined function known as an activation function. (b) Three-layer neural network.

A neural network is a massively equivalent distributed process, made up of simple processing units, which have a property for storing knowledge and making it available for use. One of the most important properties of neural networks is their ability to learn from examples; that is, learn to produce a certain output when fed with a certain input. The learning process involves modification of the connection weights, to make its overall performance correspond to a desired performance defined by the set of training examples (Figure 3.11).

For each example in the training set, there exists an input pattern and a desired output pattern. To train the network, an example from the training set is chosen and fed to the network to see what output it produces. If the expected output is not obtained, the internal weights of the network are modified according to a training algorithm, so as to minimize the difference between the desired and the actual output. The training is then continued with another training example and so on, until the network has reached steady state. Here, a fully connected network is employed and the standard backpropagation algorithm can be used for training.

3.6 SUMMARY

An EEG has a wide range of techniques through which analysis is possible to delete the unwanted noise and bring out the useful information before classifying it. Firstly, analysis of the signal is required. Fourier transform and wavelet transform are such techniques that give us an in-depth view of the content of the signal. Secondly, depending on the application, noise removal and removal of unimportant signals are implemented to take out the useful information for further processing. The techniques involved in this are wavelet denoising, band-pass filtering, median filtering, etc. Different applications require different feature extraction methods. PCA, ICA, eigenvector, and power of signal are good examples of feature extraction methods. The features that are extracted can be used for classification. Some of the popular classification techniques involved are traditional method-based classification, SVM, ANN, KNN, CNN, etc. There are other techniques that are an ongoing in the field of research. EEG signal preprocessing is one of the areas where research is being done in order to increase consistency of the signal.

Exercises

1. What different signal filtering techniques are used for processing EEG signals?
2. What is a continuous wavelet transform (CWT)? What is the output of CWT applied on an EEG signal?
3. What is Mallat's algorithm?
4. What are baseline drift phenomena in EEG signals? Explain the baseline drift removal method for EEG signals.
5. List the families of wavelet transforms.
6. What is a moving average? How does it improve the quality of EEG signals?
7. What is wavelet denoising of EEG signals? How does it improve the quality of EEG signals?
8. What are the parameters generated from FFT of EEG signals?
9. What are the parameters generated from CWT of EEG signals?
10. What are the parameters generated from discrete cosine transform of EEG signals?
11. How does ICA (independent component transform) help in source segregation of the EEG signals?
12. Discuss two prominent feature extraction techniques used for EEG signals.
13. List some of the feature classification techniques.
14. What is a SVM (support vector machine)? How does it classify EEG signals?
15. What are Hjorth parameters? How are they useful in analyzing EEG signals?

REFERENCES

Alday, PM 2019, 'How much baseline correction do we need in ERP research? Extended GLM model can replace baseline correction while lifting its limits', *Psychophysiology Journal*, 56, 12. arXiv:1707.08152v3 [stat.AP].

Al-Fahoum, AS & Al-Fraihat, AA 2014 February 13, 'Methods of EEG signal features extraction using linear analysis in frequency and time-frequency domains', *ISRN Neuroscience*, vol. 2014, p. 2014. Article ID: 730218 . doi:10.1155/2014/730218

AL-Quraishi, MS, Elamvazuthi, I, Daud, SA, Parasuraman, S & Borboni, A 2018, 'EEG-based control for upper and lower limb exoskeletons and prostheses: A systematic review', *Sensors*, vol. 18, pp. 10. http://www.mdpi.com/1424-8220/18/10/3342

Fasano, A & Villani, V 2014 June, 'Baseline wander removal for bioelectrical signals by quadratic variation reduction', *Journal Signal Processing*, vol. 99, pp. 48–57. doi: 10.1016/j.sigpro.2013.11.033

Gonzalez, RC & Wintz, P 1987, *Digital Image Processing*, Addison-Wesley, Boston, MA.

Hjorth, B & Elema-Schönander, AB 1970, 'EEG analysis based on time domain properties', *Electroencephalography and Clinical Neurophysiology*, vol. 29, pp. 306–310. doi: 10.1016/0013-4694(70)90143-4.

Isa, NEM, Amir, A, Ilyas, MZ & Razalli, MS 2017, 'The performance analysis of k-nearest neighbors (K-NN) algorithm for motor imagery classification based on EEG signal', in MATEC Web of Conferences, vol. 140, pp. 01024. doi:10.1051/matecconf/201714001024

Konstantinidis, E, Conci, N, Bamparopoulos, G, Sidiropoulos, E, De Natale, F & Bamidis, P 2015, 'Introducing neuroberry, a platform for pervasive EEG signaling in the IoT domain', *in 5th EAI International Conference on Wireless Mobile Communication and Healthcare*, London, Great Britain, 166–169. doi:10.4108/eai.14-10-2015.2261698

Lekshmi, SS, Selvam, V & Rajasekaran, MP 2014, 'EEG signal classification using principal component analysis and wavelet transform with neural network', in *2014 International Conference on Communication and Signal Processing*, Melmaruvathur, pp. 687–690. doi:10.1109/ICCSP.2014.6949930

Moghim, N & Corne, DW 2014, 'Predicting epileptic seizures in advance', *PloS one*, vol. 9, no. 6, pp. e99334. doi:10.1371/journal.pone.0099334

Paranjape, RB 2009, 'Chapter 1 – Fundamental enhancement techniques', *Handbook of Medical Image Processing and Analysis* (Second Edition), (pp. 3–18). Academic Press. ISBN 9780123739049. doi:10.1016/B978-012373904-9.50008-8

Subha, DP, Joseph, PK, Acharya UR et al. 2010, EEG signal analysis: A survey, *Journal of Medical Systems*, vol 34, p. 195. doi:10.1007/s10916-008-9231-z

Sun, L, Liu, Y & Beadle, PJ 2005, 'Independent component analysis of EEG signals', in *Proceedings of the 2005 IEEE International Workshop on VLSI Design and Video Technology, 2005*, Suzhou, China, pp. 219–222. doi:10.1109/IWVDVT.2005.1504590

4 Software and Hardware for EEG for Capturing and Analysis

OVERVIEW

This chapter analyzes the system architecture of a EEG acquisition system, which contains the hardware components, software components, and the interconnection among them. Various options for sensing the EEG signal, filtering noise, boosting the signal, aggregating the signal, and finally visualizing the EEG data are discussed. The software-specific toolboxes available for analysis of EEG data are discussed. The toolkits for visualization and analysis of EEG data available in MATLAB®, Python, and EEG lab are discussed so that a student or researcher can immediately benefit from choosing and using one of the available options for processing of EEG data for their research and experimentation.

4.1 INTRODUCTION

A typical adult human EEG signal is about 10 μV to 100 μV in amplitude when measured from the scalp and is about 10–20 μV when measured from subdural electrodes. An EEG has a very high temporal resolution, on the order of milliseconds rather than seconds. EEGs are commonly recorded at sampling rates between 250 and 2,000 Hz in clinical and research settings, but modern EEG data collection systems are capable of recording at sampling rates above 20,000 Hz if desired. Therefore, sophisticated hardware is required to acquire, amplify, denoise, and analyze the EEG signal. On searching the Internet, we found OPENBCI (https://openbci.com) is the most popular and readily available design that can be printed with 3D printers and there is also an option to buy it. Next in the list is Emotivepoc+ (https://www.emotiv.com). It comes with a wireless transaction facility and multiple channel supports. With this setup, one needs to subscribe to the interfacing software package for its operation. Next, we found an Indian manufacturer who is making medical grade EEG systems as RMSIndia (http://www.rmsindia.com/neurology.html) and Axxonet Pvt. Ltd. and used their 32-channel EEG acquisition system for our obtaining the EEG data during our experiment on various subjects (https://www.axxonet.com/medical/13-medical/27-brain-electro-scan-system-bess-eeg-erp-systems). They have 16–256-channel EEG acquisition systems. There are several open source and COTS (commercial off the shelf) EEG analysis software tools readily available for researchers and

DOI: 10.1201/9781003241386-4

the student community for processing analysis of EEG data. A couple prominent toolbox are (1) the EEGLab tool box of MATLAB and (2) the EDFLIB of Python. Some of the functions which are developed and tested for analysis of the EEG data are listed in the appendix of this book for the benefit of the students and researchers to start with.

4.2 OVERVIEW OF AN EEG SIGNAL ACQUISITION SYSTEM

Let us discuss the system with components from head electrodes to a display with the steps and processes and how the signal is amplified.

A generic block diagram depicting various components required to compose a EEG acquisition system is depicted (Figure 4.1). The various subsystems/components of the system are (a) the electrodes that are placed directly in-situ with the scalp to sense and collect the EEG signal emanating from the brain, (b) the instrumentation amplifier that amplifies the acquired EEG signal, (c) active high-pass filter and active low-pass filters that can be manifested as hardware or software components, (d) notch filter, (e) adder or aggregator (f) DAQ card, and finally (g) the subsystem for storage and display.

There are different options in component level with respect to each of these subsystems. An EEG system can have a set of compatible subsystems to compose an overall EEG acquisition system. There are many criteria for compatibility of these subsystems to acquire, process, visualize, and classify the EEG signal. The criteria and their comparison is listed in the next session.

The overall accuracy of the system depends upon the accuracy of each and every component used and their accuracy level. The optimum value of the system parameter like lead-off detection, input referred noise, CMRR, SNR, precision, etc. can be achieved with careful choice of subsystem accuracy.

A comparison of research-grade EEG acquisition systems with respect to sampling rate (Hz), number of channels, accuracy, CPU used, type of electrodes, and method of input/output (I/O), CMRR, and cost is listed in Table 4.1.

- **CMMR:** The CMRR (common mode rejection ratio) is the most important specification and it indicates how much of the common mode signals will be present to measure. The value of the CMMR frequently depends on the signal frequency and the function should be specified. (For a research-grade EEG acquisition system, the CMRR should be in the range of 90 dB–110 dB.)
- **SNR:** The best explanation of SNR is that it is the ratio of "everything you want to measure in the EEG signal" to "everything else picked up by the **EEG** signal." This noise is a problem because there are two major sources of noise inEEG signals.

  The SNR is further defined for each source location (dipole or extended patch) in decibel units computed as the signal-to-noise ratio (SNR) as a standard method to assess the signal quality. The SNR values were calculated using Equation 4.1:

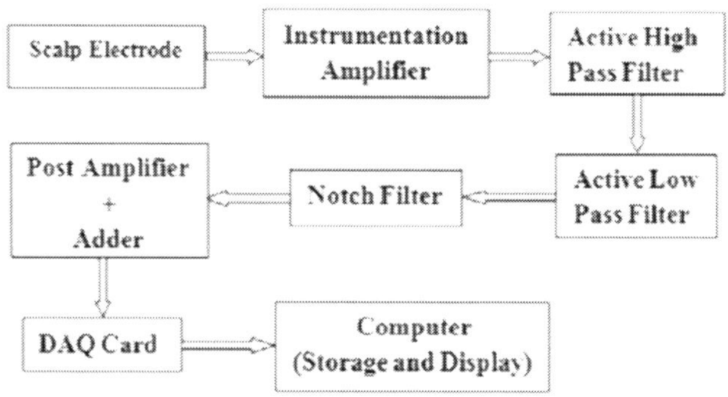

FIGURE 4.1 Generic block diagram of EEG acquisition system.

$$SNR = 10 \cdot \log_{10}(\sigma_x^2/\sigma_e^2)[\text{dB}] \tag{4.1}$$

where σ^2_x is the variance of the signal and σ^2_e is the variance of the noise. For zero mean EEG signals, the SNR is computed using Equation 4.2:

$$SNR = 10 \cdot \log_{10} \frac{\sum_{i=1}^{N} x_i^2}{\sum_{i=1}^{N} (s_i - x_i)^2} \tag{4.2}$$

where N is the number of sample points, x_i is the noise reduced signal at time i, and s_i is the band-pass filtered signal at time i. Practically, EEG SNR ranged from less than 1 dB to more than 10 dB.

4.2.1 EEG Signal Enhancement Techniques

The appropriate choice of EEG signal enhancement technique plays a crucial role in designing a EEG acquisition system. The various signal processing techniques used for enhancing the quality of the EEG signal for further processing are listed in Table 4.2. The detail processing methods are discussed in Chapter 3. In this table, we discuss the advantages and disadvantages of each of these signal enhancement techniques with respect to their capability to enhance the EEG signal so that appropriate and informed decisions can be made while choosing the processing of the acquired EEG signal.

4.2.2 Comparison of Feature Extraction Methods

Having acquired the EEG signal with appropriate signal acquisition technique, signal enhancement, signal denoising, and filtering, the EEG signal is ready for processing to extract appropriate features from the signal so that subsequent classification based on the signal feature can be taken. Table 4.3 lists and compares and contrasts various EEG feature extraction techniques.

TABLE 4.1
Comparing state-of-the-art professional BCI systems

System	Sampling Speed, Hz	Number of Channels	Accuracy	CPU	Electrodes	I/O	CMRR	Price
g.tec (https://in.mathworks.com/help/matlab/release-notes-R2014a.html)Nautilus	500	64	24-bit, <60 nV(LSB), <0.6 μVRMS	TI DSP	Active-dry/gel	Wireless 2.4GHz/USB	>90 dB	>4.5k
g.tec Hlamp	38.4k	256	24-bit, <60 nV(LSB), <0.5 μVRMS	TI DSP	Active-dry/gel	USB	>90 dB	>31k
TMSi (https://sccn.ucsd.edu/eeglab/index.php)mobita	2000	32	24-bit, <24 nV	N/A	Passive dry	Wi-Fi IEEE802.11b/g	>100 dB	N/A
TMSi (https://www.teuniz.net/edfbrowser)Porti	2048	32	22-bit, <1 μVRMS	N/A	Active-Shielding	Bluetooth/optic fiber	>90 dB	N/A
TMSi Refa	2048	136	22-bit, <1 μVRMS	N/A	Active-Shielding	Optic fiber	>90 dB	N/A

TABLE 4.2
Comparison of signal enhancement methods

Sl No.	Method	Advantages	Disadvantages
1	ICA	• Computationally efficient . • Shows high performance for large-sized data. • Decomposes signals into temporal independent and spatial fixed components.	• Can't be applicable for under-determined cases. • Requires more computations for decomposition.
2	PCA	• A powerful tool for analyzing and reducing the dimensionality of data without important loss of information.	• Assumes data is linear and continuous. • For complicated manifold, PCA fails to process data.
3	WT	• Able to analyze signal with discontinuities through variable window size. • It can analyze signals both in time and frequency domains. • Can extract energy, distance, or clusters, etc.	• Lack of specific methodology to apply WT to the pervasive noise. • Performance limited by Heisenberg uncertainty.
4	AR	• Requires only shorter duration of data records. • Reduces spectral loss problems and gives better frequency resolution.	• Difficulties exist in establishing the model properties for EEG signals. • Not applicable to non-stationary signal.
5	WPD	• Can analyze the non-stationary signals.	• Increased computation time.
6	FFT	• Powerful method of frequency analysis.	• Applicable only to stationary signals and linear random processes. • Suffers from large noise sensitivity. • Poor time localization makes it not suitable to all kinds of applications.

4.2.3 EEG Signal Classification Methods

Having extracted the features from the acquired EEG, an appropriate signal classification method is required for classification of the features of the acquired EEG signal. In Table 4.4, some of the important classification methods used frequently are listed. Also, we discuss the advantages and disadvantages of these EEG signal classification methods so that an appropriate decision can be made for composition of the overall EEG acquisition system.

TABLE 4.3
Comparison of feature extraction methods

Sl No.	Method	Advantages	Disadvantages
1	ICA	• Computationally efficient. • Shows high performance for large-sized data. • Decomposes signals into temporal independent and spatial fixed components.	• Can't be appliable for under-determined cases. • Require more computations for decomposition.
2	CAR	• Outperforms all the reference methods. • Yields improved SNR.	• Finite sample density and incomplete head coverage cause problems in calculating averages.
3	SL	• Robust against the artifacts generated at regions that are not covered by electrode cap. • It solves electrode reference problem.	• Sensitive to artifacts. • Sensitive to spline patterns.
4	PCA	• Helps in reduction of feature dimensions. • Ranking will be done and helps in classification of data.	• Not as well as ICA.
5	CSP	• Doesn't require a priori selection of subspecific bands and knowledge of these bands.	• Requires use of many electrodes. • Change in position of electrode may affect classification accuracies.
6	Adaptive filtering	• Ability to modify the signal features according to signals is being analyzed. • Works well for the signals and artifacts with overlapping spectra nature.	

4.3 EEG ACQUISITION: AXXONET'S BRAIN ELECTRO SCAN SYSTEM (BESS)

Having been developed for research purposes, BESS is equipped with a user-friendly stimulus presentation package, capable of presenting stimuli in visual and auditory modality, with unique provisions for customizing its stimulus presentation properties (https://www.axxonet.com/medical/13-medical/27-brain-electro-scan-system-bess-eeg-erp-systems),(https://www.youtube.com/watch?v=BX3MG2yFBuY).

TABLE 4.4
EEG signal classification methods

Sl No.	Method	Advantages	Disadvantages
1	LDA	• It has low computational requirements. • Simple to use. • It provides good results.	• It fails when the discriminatory function not in mean but in variance of the features. • For non-Gaussian distributions it may not preserve the complex structures.
2	SVM	• It provides good generalization. • Performance is more than other linear classifier.	• Has high computational complexity.
3	ANN	• Ease of use and implementation. • Robust in nature. • Simple computations are involved. • Small training set requirements are required. • Small training set requirements are required.	• Difficult to build. • Performance depends on the number of neutrons in hidden layer.
4	NBC	• Requires only a small amount of training data to estimate parameters. • Only variance of class variables is to be computed and no need to compute the entire covariance matrix.	• Fails to produce a good estimate for the correct class probabilities.
5	K-NN	• Very simple to understand. • Easy to implement and debug.	• Poor runtime performance if training set is large. • Sensitive to irrelevant and redundant features. • On difficult classification tasks, outperformed by other classification methods.

- BESS provides a comprehensive stimulus presentation package that automates functions related to ERP presentation from presentation to analysis, the first of its kind. *In addition, BESS interfaces with tools such as E-Prime and Open Sesame.*
- The xAmp series of amplifiers have 8 to 128 channels and 24-bit resolution with simultaneous sampling of 20 KHz per channel in select models. With a low noise floor of <1 μV, the xAmp series ensures high-quality recordings.
- xAmp can interface with third-party headsets and headgear including active electrodes.

- xAmp has direct interfaces with Axxonet's innovative Rapid Cap, the new ultra-fast deployment multi-contact EEG cap that supports saline and gel recordings.
- BESS has built-in digital EEG data processing capabilities that are complex, yet accurate and only found in solutions like Octave or MATLAB.
- Its advanced analysis package makes BESS a complete and one of the finest ERP tools for research in the area of neuroscience, be it cognitive science, neuropsychology, or electrophysiology.
- BESS is a highly sophisticated, user-friendly system developed for acquisition and analysis of bioelectrical brain activity.
- It is employed in research under neuroscience, cognitive psychology, cognitive science, and psycho-physiology. It is available in auditory and visual modalities.
- The systems are highly accurate with complex data processing and analysis capabilities. The systems are built over years of research and development in the field of electroencephalography.
- BESS is available in desktop and laptop versions for mobile recordings.
- BESS models are available in 16-, 32-, 64-, 128-, and 256-channel configurations and can be built customized per requirements.
- Provisions are available to customize it as per the requirement for clinical application and diagnosis as well (Figure 4.2).

- **EEG – ERP Recordings**
  - Ability to treat each stimulus as an event with additional keyboard events
  - Ability to mark beginnings and end of stimulus, pre-stimulus duration
  - Group batch of stimulus into bins
  - Edit event makers and save as a new file

The BESS clinical models are available in 16-, 32-, 64-, 128-, and 256-channel configurations and can be built customized per requirements. The systems are available in desktop versions and laptop versions.

4.4 SOFTWARE REQUIREMENT FOR ANALYZING EEGS

4.4.1 MATLAB

MATLAB® (https://in.mathworks.com/help/matlab/release-notes-R2014a.html) is the high-level language and interactive environment used by millions of engineers and scientists worldwide. It lets one explore and visualize ideas and collaborate across disciplines including signal and image processing, communications, control systems, and computational finance. MATLAB can be used to run millions of simulations to pinpoint optimal dosing for antibiotics.

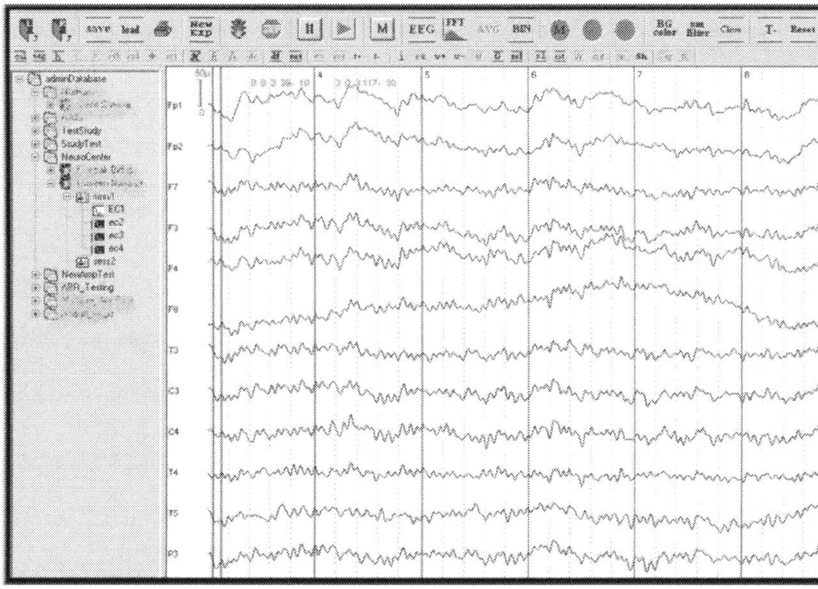

FIGURE 4.2 EEG acquisition in real time using BESS.

MATLAB is a high-performance language for technical computing. It integrates computation, visualization, and programming in an easy-to-use environment where problems and solutions are expressed in familiar mathematical notation. Typical uses include math and computation and signal processing. In the context of EEG signal processing, the signal processing toolbox provided by MATLAB is of special importance to build different filters and feature extraction tools.

The Signal Processing Toolbox™ provides functions and apps to analyze, pre-process, and extract features from uniformly and non-uniformly sampled signals. With the filter designer app, one can design and analyze digital filters by choosing from a variety of algorithms and responses.

4.4.1.1 Key Features of MATLAB

- High-level language for numerical computation, visualization, and application development
- Interactive environment for iterative exploration, design, and problem solving
- Mathematical functions for linear algebra, statistics, Fourier analysis, filtering, optimization, numerical integration, and solving ordinary differential equations
- Built-in graphics for visualizing data and tools for creating custom plots
- Development tools for improving code quality and maintainability and maximizing performance

- Tools for building applications with custom graphical interfaces
- Functions for integrating MATLAB-based algorithms with external applications and languages such as C, Java, NET, and Microsoft® Excel for further computing, analysis, and visualization of the EEG artifacts.

4.4.1.2 Functions

Numeric computation MATLAB provides a range of numerical computation methods for analyzing data, developing algorithms, and creating models. The MATLAB language includes mathematical functions that support common engineering and science operations. Core math functions use processor-optimized libraries to provide fast execution of vector and matrix calculations.

- **Available Methods Include:**
  1. Interpolation and regression
  2. Differentiation and integration
  3. Linear systems of equations
  4. Fourier analysis
  5. Eigen values and singular values
  6. Ordinary differential equations (ODEs)
  7. Sparse matrices
  8. Wavelet analysis

4.4.1.3 Data Analysis and Visualization

MATLAB provides tools to acquire, analyze, and visualize data, enabling one to gain insight into the data in a fraction of the time it would take using spreadsheets or traditional programming languages. One can also document and share the results through plots and reports or as published MATLAB code.

4.4.1.4 Acquiring Data

MATLAB lets one access data from files, other applications, databases, and external devices. One can read data from popular file formats such as Microsoft Excel; text or binary files; image, sound, and video files; and scientific files such as net, CDF, and HDF. File I/O functions let one work with data files in any format. Using MATLAB with add-on products, one can acquire data from hardware devices, such as your computer's serial port or sound card, as well as stream live, measured data directly into MATLAB for analysis and visualization. One can also communicate with instruments such as oscilloscopes, function generators, and signal analyzers.

4.4.1.5 Analyzing Data

MATLAB lets one manage, filter, and pre-process the data. One can perform exploratory data analysis to uncover trends, test assumptions, and build descriptive models. MATLAB provides functions for filtering and smoothing, interpolation, convolution, and fast Fourier transforms (FFTs). Add-on products provide capabilities for curve and surface fitting, multivariate statistics, spectral analysis, image analysis, system identification, and other analysis tasks.

4.4.1.6 Visualizing Data

MATLAB provides built-in 2D and 3D plotting functions, as well as volume visualization functions. One can use these functions to visualize and understand data and communicate results. Plots can be customized either interactively or programmatically. The MATLAB plot gallery provides examples of many ways to display data graphically in MATLAB. For each example, one can view and download source code to use in the MATLAB application.

4.4.1.7 Documenting and Sharing Results

One can share results as plots or complete reports. MATLAB plots can be customized to meet publication specifications and saved to common graphical and data file formats. One can automatically generate a report when one executes a MATLAB program. The report contains the code, comments, and program results, including plots. Reports can be published in a variety of formats, such as HTML, PDF, Word, or LaTeX.

4.4.1.8 Programming and Algorithm Development

MATLAB provides high-level language and development tools that let one quickly develop and analyze algorithms and applications.

4.4.1.9 Application Development and Deployment

MATLAB tools and add-on products provide a range of options to develop and deploy applications. One can share individual algorithms and applications with other MATLAB users or deploy them royalty-free to others who do not have MATLAB.

4.4.1.10 Designing Graphic User Interface

Using GUIDE (Graphical User Interface Development Environment), one can lay out, design, and edit custom graphical user interfaces. One can include common controls such as list boxes, pull-down menus, and push buttons, as well as MATLAB plots. Graphical user interfaces can also be created programmatically using MATLAB functions.

4.4.1.11 Generating C Code

One can use MATLAB Coder to generate stand-alone C code from MATLAB code. MATLAB Coder supports a subset of the MATLAB language typically used by design engineers for developing algorithms as components of larger systems. This code can be used for stand-alone execution, for integration with other software applications, or as part of an embedded application.

4.4.1.12 Development Tools

MATLAB includes a variety of tools for efficient algorithm development, including:

1. **Command Window:** Lets you interactively enter data, execute commands and programs, and display results.
2. **MATLAB Editor:** Provides editing and debugging features, such as setting break points and stepping through individual lines of code.
3. **Code Analyzer:** Automatically checks code for problems and recommends modifications to maximize performance and maintainability.
4. **MATLAB Profiler:** Measures performance of MATLAB programs and identifies areas of code to modify for improvement.

4.4.1.13 Syntax

The MATLAB application is built around the MATLAB language, and most of MATLAB involves typing MATLAB code into the Command Window (as an interactive mathematical shell), or executing text files containing MATLAB code, including scripts and/or functions.

4.4.1.14 Variables

Variables are defined using the assignment operator, "=" in MATLAB is a weekly typed programming language because types are implicitly converted. It is an inferred typed language because variables can be assigned without declaring their type, except if they are to be treated as symbolic objects, and their type can change. Values can come from constants, from computation involving values of other variables, or from the output of a function.

4.4.1.15 Matrices

Matrices can be defined by separating the elements of a row with a blank space or comma and using a semicolon to terminate each row. The list of elements should be surrounded by square brackets: []. Parentheses () are used to access elements and sub-arrays (they are also used to denote a function argument list).

4.4.1.16 Structures

MATLAB has structure data types. Since all variables in MATLAB are arrays, a more adequate name is "structure array," where each element of the array has the same field names. In addition, MATLAB supports dynamic field names (field look-ups by name, field manipulations, etc.). Unfortunately, MATLAB JIT does not support MATLAB structures; therefore, just a simple bundling of various variables into a structure will come at a cost.

4.4.1.17 GUI Programming

MATLAB supports developing applications with graphical user interface features. MATLAB includes GUIDE (GUI development environment) for graphically designing GUIs. It also has tightly integrated graph-plotting features.

4.4.1.18 Applications

1. Data exploration, acquisition, analyzing, and visualization
2. Engineering drawing and scientific graphics

3. Analyzing algorithmic designing and development
4. Mathematical functions and computational functions
5. Simulating problems, prototyping, and modeling
6. Application development programming using GUI building environment

4.5 EEGLAB TOOLBOX

An EEG signal is saved in European Data Format (.edf), which cannot be opened directly in MATLAB. The EEGLAB (https://sccn.ucsd.edu/eeglab/index.php) toolbox provides support for reading different formats of EEG files and plots them by analyzing different useful in-built functions. EEGLAB is an interactive MATLAB toolbox for processing continuous and event-related EEG, MEG, and other electrophysiological data incorporating independent component analysis (ICA), time/frequency analysis, artifact rejection, event-related statistics, and several useful modes of visualization of the averaged and single-trial data. EEGLAB runs under Linux, Unix, Windows, and Mac OS.

EEGLAB provides an interactive graphic user interface (GUI), allowing users to flexibly and interactively process their high-density EEG and other dynamic brain data using independent component analysis (ICA) and/or time/frequency analysis (TFA), as well as standard averaging methods. It also incorporates extensive tutorial and help windows, plus a command history function that eases users' transition from GUI-based data exploration to building and running batch or custom data analysis scripts. EEGLAB offers a wealth of methods for visualizing and modeling event-related brain dynamics, both at the level of individual EEGLAB "data sets" and/or across a collection of data sets brought together in an EEGLAB "study set."

For experienced MATLAB users, EEGLAB offers a structured programming environment for storing, accessing, measuring, manipulating, and visualizing event-related EEG data. For creative research programmers and methods developers, EEGLAB offers an extensible, open-source platform through which they can share new methods with the world research community by publishing EEGLAB "plug-in" functions that appear automatically in the EEGLAB menu of users who download them. For example, novel EEGLAB plug-ins might be built and released to "pick peaks" in ERP or time/frequency results, or to perform specialized import/export, data visualization, or inverse source modeling of EEG, MEG, and/or ECOG data. Figure 4.3 demonstrates the EEGLAB GUI window opened in MATLAB.

4.5.1 EEGLAB Features

- Graphic user interface
- Multi-format data importing
- High-density data scrolling
- Interactive plotting functions
- Semi-automated artifact removal
- ICA and time/frequency transforms

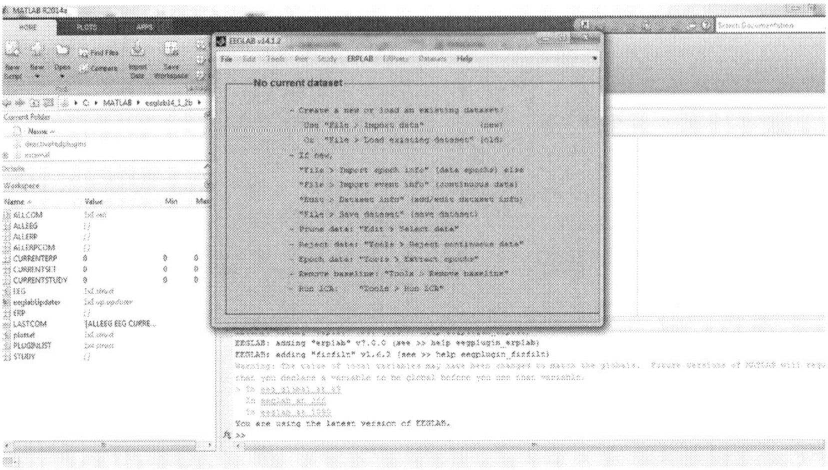

FIGURE 4.3 EEG LAB GUI window in MATLAB.

- Event and channel location handling
- Forward/inverse head/source modeling
- Defined EEG data structure
- Many advanced plug-in/extension toolboxes

4.5.2 EEGLAB System Requirements

- **MATLAB version:** The latest version of EEGLAB runs on MATLAB 7.6 (2008b) or later under any operating system (Linux/Unix, Windows, Mac OSX). For earlier MATLAB versions, download the legacy version EEGLAB v4.3, which will run on MATLAB 5.3. EEGLAB extensions (in particular BCILAB and SIFT) also require MATLAB 7.6 or later. Note that all EEGLAB signal processing functions also run on the free MATLAB clone Octave, although graphics cannot be displayed (this is useful for high-performance computing applications – see the EEGLAB wiki for more details).
- **Memory requirements:** Using multi-core 64-bit processors with large amounts of RAM may be essential for analyzing large data sets – 8 Gb or more RAM is recommended (also see the EEGLAB wiki tutorial for tips on minimizing memory usage). Linux is preferred as an environment for processing EEG data using EEGLAB, mostly because of better memory management of MATLAB under Linux (if using Linux, choose Fedora over Ubuntu as there are sometimes minor graphics problem with how MATLAB handles OpenGL under Ubuntu).
- **Additional MATLAB toolboxes:** EEGLAB requires no additional toolboxes. However, some toolboxes are recommended. By order of importance:

- **Signal processing toolbox:** Although EEGLAB incorporates functions to replace functions it uses from this toolbox when necessary (e.g., for filtering and power spectra computation), they are not as efficient as the toolbox MATLAB functions. This toolbox is also required by some EEGLAB extensions such as SIFT. This is probably the most important toolbox to have.
- **Statistics toolbox:** This toolbox is required by some EEGLAB extensions (such as Fieldtrip and SIFT). This toolbox also contains a large number of functions useful for the advanced programmer to compute statistics and cross-validation.
- **Optimization toolbox:** This is another recommended toolbox used by some EEGLAB extensions. This toolbox contains the powerful fminsearch function and derivative. Although MATLAB now has this function by default in its core distribution, the optimization toolbox allows performing finer tuning of its parameters.
- **Image processing toolbox:** This toolbox is required by some EEGLAB extensions (such as Fieldtrip).

- **Post-processing:** After figures are exported in the postscript vector format from MATLAB/EEGLAB, a postscript editor is usually necessary to fine-tune them for publication.

4.6 EDF BROWSER

EDF browser is a free, open-source, multiplatform, universal viewer and toolbox intended for, but not limited to, time series storage files like EEG, EMG, ECG, Bio-Impedance, etc. (https://www.teuniz.net/edfbrowser). EDF browser is a very helpful tool to visualize events in EEG recordings with the option to play video recorded during the session (Figure 4.4). It combines with a VLC player to do the previously mentioned options.

4.6.1 EDF Browser Features

- Easy to install, just one executable, no special requirements, no Octave or MATLAB needed
- EDF browser is one of the fastest, if not the fastest, EDF viewer available (Figure 4.4)
- Supported file formats: EDF, EDF+, BDF, BDF+
- Nihon Kohden (*.eeg) to EDF+ converter (including annotations)
- Unisens to EDF+ converter
- MIT to EDF+ converter (including annotations) for Physiobank
- ManscanMicroamps (*.mbi/*.mb2) to EDF+ converter (including annotations)
- SCP-ECG (*.scp, EN 1064) to EDF+ converter
- Synchronous video playback

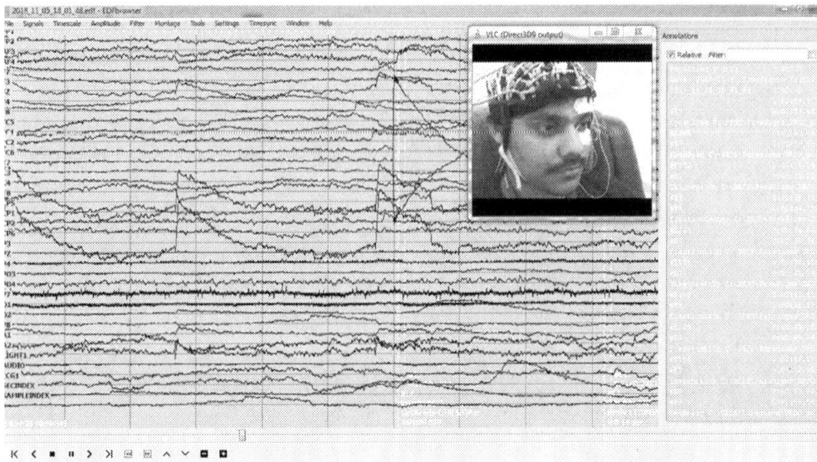

FIGURE 4.4 Visualizing a recording session with EDF browser.

- Emsa (*.PLG) to EDF+ converter (including annotations)
- ASCII to EDF/BDF converter
- Finometer (Beatscope) to EDF converter
- Bmeye Nexfin (FrameInspector) to EDF converter
- WAV to EDF converter
- Mortara XML ECG to EDF converter
- Reads Biosemi's trigger inputs from the BDF "Status" signal
- Annotation editor
- Header editor, fixes also lots of different format errors
- 1st to 8th order Butterworth, Chebyshev, Bessel, and "moving average" filters
- Notch filter with adjustable Q-factor
- Customizable FIR filter
- Spike filter removes spikes, glitches, fast transients, or pacemaker impulses
- Power spectrum (FFT)
- ECG heart rate detection (raw ECG waveform -> beats per minute)
- With possibility to export the RR-intervals (beat to beat)
- FM modulated (transtelephonic) ECG recording to EDF converter
- Z-EEG measurement
- Averaging using triggers, events, or annotations
- Supports montages
- Annotations/events export
- Annotations/events import
- File reducer/cropper/decimator
- Down sampling signals
- Precise measurements by using crosshairs

- Zoom function by drawing a rectangle with the mouse
- Shows signals from different files at the same time
- EDF/EDF+/BDF/BDF+ to ASCII converter
- EDF/EDF+/BDF/BDF+ compatibility checker
- EDF+D to EDF+C converter
- BDF (+) to EDF (+) converter
- Prints to a printer, image, or PDF
- Combines several files and exports it to one new EDF file
- Exports part of a file to a new file
- Reads from a streaming file (monitor)
- Available for Linux and Windows (the source can be compiled on Mac OS X)

4.7 PYTHON

Python is a general-purpose interpreted, interactive, object-oriented, and high-level programming language. It was created by Guido van Rossum during 1985–1990. Like Perl, Python source code is also available under the GNU General Public License (GPL). Python's design philosophy emphasizes code readability with its notable use of significant white space. Its language constructs and object-oriented approach aims to help programmers write clear, logical code for small and large-scale projects (Kuhlman 2012). Van Rossum shouldered sole responsibility for the project until July 2018, but now shares his leadership as a member of a five-person steering council. Figure 4.5 shows a Python terminal window.

4.7.1 Python Features

Python's features include:

- **Easy to learn:** Python has few keywords, simple structure, and a clearly defined syntax. This allows the student to pick up the language quickly.

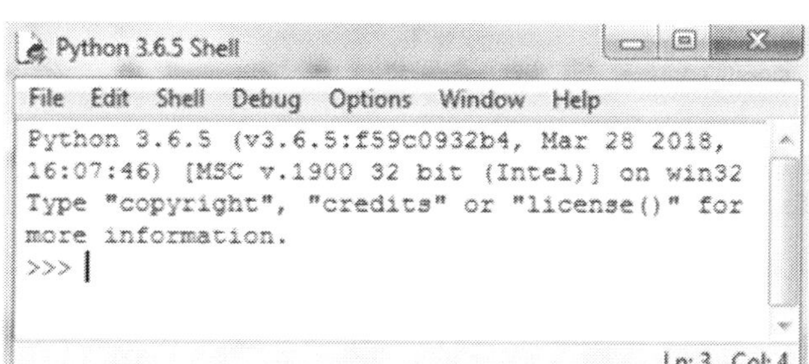

FIGURE 4.5 Python shell terminal.

- **Easy to read:** Python code is more clearly defined and visible to the eyes.
- **Easy to maintain:** Python's source code is fairly easy to maintain.
- **A broad standard library:** Python's bulk of the library is very portable and cross-platform compatible on UNIX, Windows, and Macintosh.
- **Interactive mode:** Python has support for an interactive mode that allows interactive testing and debugging of snippets of code.
- **Portable:** Python can run on a wide variety of hardware platforms and has the same interface on all platforms.
- **Extendable:** One can add low-level modules to the Python interpreter. These modules enable programmers to add to or customize their tools to be more efficient.
- **Databases:** Python provides interfaces to all major commercial databases.
- **GUI programming:** Python supports GUI applications that can be created and ported to many system calls, libraries, and windows systems, such as Windows MFC, Macintosh, and the X Window system of Unix.
- **Scalable:** Python provides a better structure and support for large programs than shell scripting.

Apart from the above-mentioned features, Python has a big list of good features, a few of which are listed below:

- It supports functional and structured programming methods as well as OOP.
- It can be used as a scripting language or can be compiled to byte-code for building large applications.
- It provides very high-level dynamic data types and supports dynamic type checking.
- It supports automatic garbage collection.
- It can be easily integrated with C, C++, COM, ActiveX, CORBA, and Java.

4.7.2 Relevant Libraries in Python

4.7.2.1 pyEDFlib

pyEDFlib is a Python library to read/write EDF+/BDF+ files based on EDFlib (https://pypi.org/project/pyEDFlib/). EDF means European Data Format and was firstly published by Kemp (1992). In 2003, an improved version of the file protocol named EDF+ has been published and (Kemp 2003).

European Data Format (EDF) is a standard file format designed for exchange and storage of medical time series. Being an open and non-proprietary format, EDF(+) is commonly used to archive, exchange, and analyze data from commercial devices in a format that is independent of the acquisition system.

The EDF/EDF+ format saves all data with 16 bits. A version that saves all data with 24 bits, was introduced by the company BioSemi.

The definition of the EDF/EDF+/BDF/BDF+ format can be found under edfplus.info.

This Python toolbox is a fork of the toolbox from Christopher Lee-Messer and uses the EDFlib from Teunis van Beelen. The EDFlib is able to read and write EDF/EDF+/BDF/BDF+ files.

4.7.2.1.1 Documentation

Documentation is available online at http://pyedflib.readthedocs.org

Process to install pyEDFlibation

pyEDFlib can be used with Python version 2.7.x or >=3.4. It depends on the NumPy package. To use the newest source code from git, you have to download the source code. One needs a C compiler and a recent version of Cython. Go to the source directory and type:

```
python setup.py build
python setup.py install
```

There are binary wheels that can be installed by:

```
pip install pyEDFlib
```

Users of the Anaconda Python distribution can directly obtain pre-built Windows, Intel Linux, or macOS/OSX binaries from the conda-forge channel. This can be done via:

```
conda install -c conda-forge pyedflib
```

The most recent development version can be found on GitHub at https://github.com/holgern/pyedflib.The latest release, including source and binary packages for Linux, macOS, and Windows, is available for download from the Python Package Index. One can find source releases on the Releases page. pyEDFlib is free, open-source software released under the BSD 2-clause license.

4.7.2.2 NumPy

NumPy is the fundamental package for scientific computing with Python (https://www.numpy.or). It contains among other things:

- A powerful N-dimensional array object
- Sophisticated (broadcasting) functions
- Tools for integrating C/C++ and Fortran code
- Useful linear algebra, Fourier transform, and random number capabilities

Besides its obvious scientific uses, NumPy can also be used as an efficient multidimensional container of generic data. Arbitrary data types can be defined. This allows NumPy to seamlessly and speedily integrate with a wide variety of databases. NumPy is licensed under the BSD license, enabling reuse with few restrictions.

4.7.2.2.1 Getting Started

To install NumPy, we strongly recommend using a *scientific Python distribution*. See Installing the SciPy Stack for details. Many high-quality online tutorials, courses, and books are available to get started with NumPy. We also recommend the SciPy Lecture Notes for a broader introduction to the scientific Python ecosystem. For more information on the SciPy Stack (for which NumPy provides the fundamental array data structure), see scipy.org.

4.7.2.2.2 Documentation

The most up-to-date NumPy documentation can be found in the latest (development) version. It includes a user guide, full reference documentation, a developer guide, meta information, and "NumPy Enhancement Proposals" (which include the NumPy Roadmap and detailed plans for major new features).

A complete archive of documentation for all NumPy releases (minor versions; bug fix releases don't contain significant documentation changes) since 2009 can be found at https://docs.scipy.org.

4.8 SUMMARY

The previously mentioned tools are highly sophisticated and recommended for EEG-related studies. Although there are a lot of resources available over the Internet, Biosig, Bio-electromagnetism, Fieldtrip, Brainstorm, Brain Vision Analyzer, etc. are preferable tools for analyzing EEG data using MATLAB; whereas in Python one can use PYEEG, MNE tools, Neuropy, etc. Most of these tools are open source. The MNE tools website has a lot of experimental EEG data available to download to give a head start.

Exercises

1. Give a block diagram describing the overall architecture of the EEG acquisition system. Give a brief note on each of its subsystems and their permissible metric measures.
2. What are the overall good metric measures of a subsystem required for building an EEG acquisition system?
3. What is CMRR? Give its permissible value for an EEG system.
4. What is SNR? Give its practical limits for an EEG system.
5. List various EEG signal enhancement techniques. Compare and contrast these techniques, describing their advantages and disadvantages.
6. List various EEG denoising techniques.

7. List various EEG feature extraction techniques.
8. List various EEG classification techniques, and discuss their advantages and disadvantages.
9. List different storage formats for EEG signals.
10. List some of the popular tools for visualization of EEG signals. Also, discuss their main functions.

REFERENCES

https://www.emotiv.com
https://health.axxonet.com
https://in.mathworks.com/help/matlab/release-notes-R2014a.html
Kuhlman, D 2012, *A Python Book: Beginning Python, Advanced Python, and Python Exercises*. Section 1.1. Archived from the original (PDF) on 23 June 2012.
https://www.numpy.or
http://openbci.com
https://pypi.org/project/pyEDFlib/
http://www.rmsindia.com/neurology.html
https://sccn.ucsd.edu/eeglab/index.php
https://www.teuniz.net/edfbrowser
https://www.youtube.com/watch?v=BX3MG2yFBuY

5 Protocol and Process of EEG Data Acquisition

OVERVIEW

This chapter discusses different topologies or the placement system of EEG electrodes on the scalp. The various standards for placement of electrodes and their indexing to refer and correlate EEG signals with the functional part of the brain are discussed. Further, the clinical protocol followed to prepare a human subject for acquisition of EEG data is discussed. The process of affixing the EEG sensor to the skull of the subject along with the EEG acquisition setup is described in a step-wise manner. Also discussed is the experimental setup so as to elicit various EEG signal artifacts for study of different behaviors of the subject.

5.1 INTRODUCTION

The first recording of the electric field of the human brain was made by the German psychiatrist Hans Berger in 1924 in Jena. He gave this recording the name electroencephalogram (EEG) (Berger 1929). (From 1929 to 1938, he published 20 scientific papers on the EEG under the same title "Über das Elektroenkephalogram des Menschen."). Since then, the EEG data can be acquired for different diagnosis purposes. Following are the main types of EEG signals acquired:

1. Spontaneous activity
2. Evoked potentials
3. Bioelectric events produced by individual neurons

Spontaneous activity is measured on the scalp or on the brain and is called the electroencephalogram. The amplitude of the EEG is about 100 μV when measured on the scalp, and about 1–2 μV when measured on the surface of the brain. The frequency bandwidth of this signal is in the range of 1 Hz to about 50 Hz.

As depicted in Figure 5.1, the phase and amplitude of the EEG signal varies continuously, implying "spontaneous and continuous activity," in the living individual.

Evoked potentials are those components of the EEG that arise in response to a stimulus (which may be electric, auditory, visual, etc.). Such signals are usually below the noise level and thus not readily distinguished. One must use a train of stimuli to the subject and perform signal processing such as signal averaging to improve the signal-to-noise ratio before analysis of the evoke potential.

DOI: 10.1201/9781003241386-5

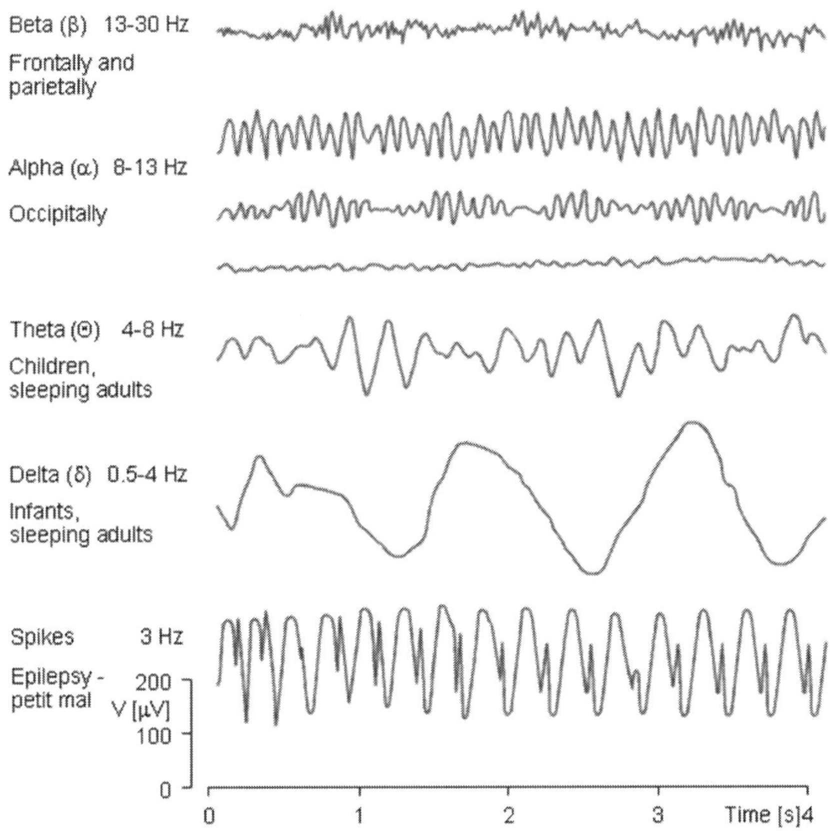

FIGURE 5.1 Different waveforms of EEG signal.

Single-neuron behavior can be examined through the use of microelectrodes that impale the cells of interest. Through studies of the single cell, one hopes to build models of neural networks or network of neurons that can reveal the actual tissue properties and brain paths among various functional parts of the brain.

Further, the behavior of the EEG signals can be differentiated as alpha (α), beta (β), delta (δ), and theta (Θ) waves as well as spikes associated with epilepsy or any neural disorder. The waveform of each class of EEG signal is depicted in Figure 5.1.

The alpha waves have the frequency spectrum of 8–13 Hz and can be measured from the occipital region in an awake state of a person when the eyes are closed. The frequency band of the beta waves is 13–30 Hz; these are detectable over the parietal and frontal lobes. The delta waves have the frequency range of 0.5–4 Hz and are detectable in infants and sleeping adults. The theta waves have the frequency range of 4–8 Hz and are obtained from children and sleeping adults.

5.2 THE BASIC PRINCIPLES OF EEG DIAGNOSIS

The EEG signal is closely related to the level of consciousness of the person. As the activity increases, the EEG shifts to a higher dominating frequency and lower amplitude. When the eyes are closed, the alpha waves begin to dominate the EEG. When the person falls asleep, the dominant EEG frequency decreases. In a certain phase of sleep, rapid eye movement (REM), the person dreams and has active movements of the eyes, which can be seen as a characteristic EEG signal. In deep sleep, the EEG has large and slow deflections called delta waves. No cerebral activity can be detected from a patient with complete cerebral death. An example of each of the mentioned waveforms is depicted in Figure 5.2.

5.3 THE EEG ELECTRODE PLACEMENT SYSTEMS

Quality of diagnosis from the EEG data depends upon proper acquisition of EEG data from the subject. This calls for choice of appropriate EEG acquisition system with standard electrode configuration and spatial placement on the scalp i.e., its spatial positioning and density. Following are the different EEG electrode placement systems and their alpha-numeric naming convention.

The international 10–20 electrode placement system uses 21 electrodes, as depicted in Figure 5.3a, b. It is an internationally recognized method to describe and apply the location of scalp electrodes in the context of an EEG acquisition from the subject. The EEG signal can be analyzed for the polysomnograph sleep study, or voluntary lab research such as detection of lie or for interfacing with any device. This method was developed to maintain standardized testing methods, ensuring that a subject's study outcomes (clinical or research) could be compiled, reproduced, and effectively analyzed and compared using the scientific method. The system is based on the relationship between the location of an electrode and the underlying area of the brain, specifically the cerebral cortex.

During sleep and wake cycles, the brain produces different, but objectively recognized and distinguishable electrical patterns. This can be can be detected by electrodes on the scalp. (These patterns might vary, and can be affected by multiple extrinsic factors, i.e., age, prescription drugs, somatic diagnoses, result of neurologic insults/injury/trauma, and substance abuse.)

The "10" and "20" refer to the fact that the actual distances between adjacent electrodes are either 10% or 20% of the total front–back or right–left distance of the skull. For example, a measurement is taken across the top of the head, from the nasion to inion. Most other common measurements ("landmarking methods") start at one ear and end at the other, normally over the top of the head. Specific anatomical locations of the ear used include the tragus, the auricle, and the mastoid.

Designating the electrodes through an alpha-numeric indexing is important so that the signals acquired can be mapped to various regions of the brain. This will make it easy to directly map the signal behavior to different regions of the brain.

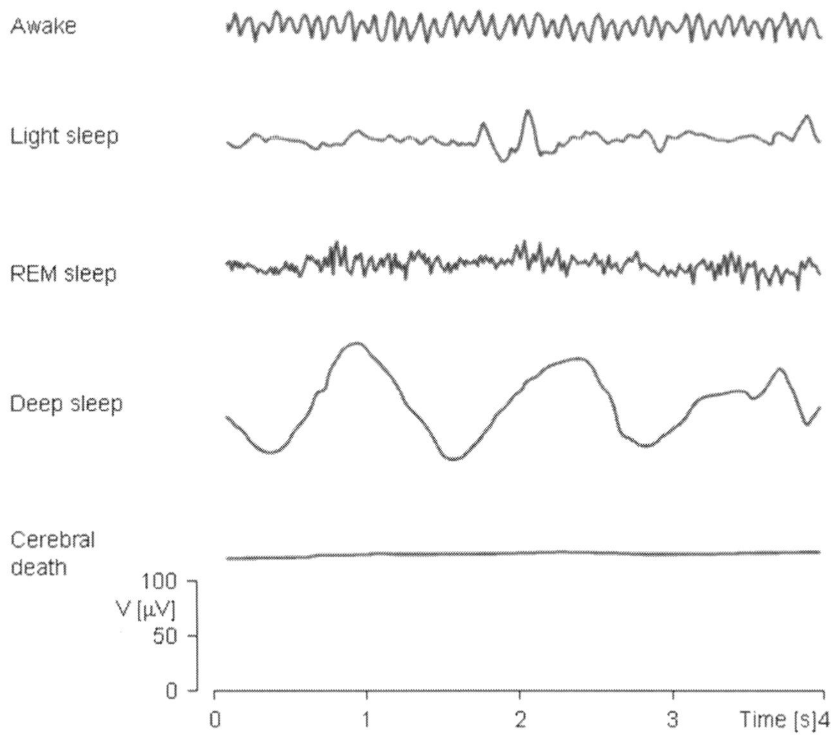

FIGURE 5.2 Waveforms of EEG signals at different levels of consciousness.

Each electrode placement site has a letter to identify the brain lobe, or area of the brain it is reading the signal from: pre-frontal (Fp), frontal (F), temporal (T), parietal (P), occipital (O), and central (C). Note that there is no "central lobe"; due to their placement, and depending on the individual, the "C" electrodes can exhibit/represent EEG activity more typical of frontal, temporal, and some parietal-occipital activity, and are always utilized in polysomnography sleep studies for the purpose of determining stages of sleep.

There are also (Z) sites: A "Z" (zero) refers to an electrode placed on the midline sagittal plane of the skull (FpZ, Fz, Cz, Oz) and is present mostly for reference/measurement points. These electrodes will not necessarily reflect or amplify lateral hemispheric cortical activity as they are placed over the corpus callosum, and do not represent either hemisphere adequately. "Z" electrodes are often utilized as "grounds" or "references," especially in polysomnography sleep studies, and diagnostic/clinical EEG montages meant to represent/diagnose epileptiform seizure activity, or possible clinical brain death. Note that the required number of EEG electrodes, and their careful, measured placement, increases with each clinical requirement and modality.

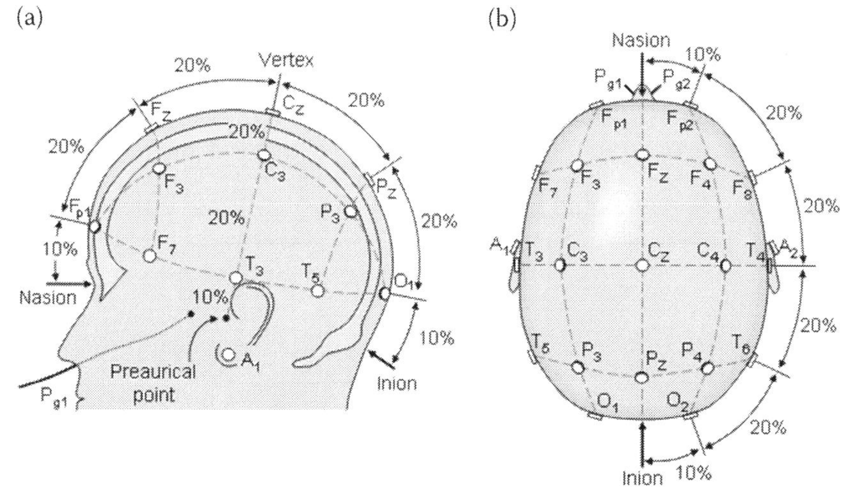

FIGURE 5.3 The international 10–20 system seen from (a) left and (b) above the head. A = ear lobe, C = central, Pg = nasopharyngeal, P = parietal, F = frontal, Fp = frontal polar, O = occipital, T= Temporal.

Conventionally, the even-numbered electrodes (2, 4, 6, 8) refer to electrode placement on the right side of the head, whereas odd numbers (1, 3, 5, 7) refer to those on the left; this applies to both EEG and EOG (electrooculogram measurements of the eye) electrodes, as well as ECG (electrocardiography measurements of the heart) electrode placement. Chin, or EMG (electromyogram) electrodes are more commonly just referred to with "right," "left," and "reference," or "common," as there are usually only three placed, and they can be differentially referenced from the EEG and EOG reference sites.

The "A" (sometimes referred to as "M" for mastoid process) refers to the prominent bone process usually found just behind the outer ear (less prominent in children and some adults). In basic polysomnography, F3, F4, Fz, Cz, C3, C4, O1, O2, A1, and A2 (M1, M2), are used. Cz and Fz are "ground" or "common" reference points for all EEG and EOG electrodes, and A1–A2 are used for contralateral referencing of all EEG electrodes. This EEG montage may be extended to utilize T3–T4, P3–P4, as well as others, if an extended or "seizure montage" is called for.

5.4 MEASUREMENT

Specific anatomical landmarks are used for the essential measuring and positioning of the EEG electrodes. These are found with a tape measure, and often marked with a grease pencil, or "China marker."

- Nasion to inion: the nasion is the distinctly depressed area between the eyes, just above the bridge of the nose, and the inion is the crest point of the back of the skull, often indicated by a bump (the prominent occipital ridge, can usually be located with mild palpation). Marks for the Z electrodes are made between these points along the midline, at intervals of 10%, 20%, 20%, 20%, 20%, and 10%.

- Preauricular to preauricular (or tragus to tragus: the tragus refers to the small portion of cartilage projecting anteriorly to the pinna). The preauricural point is in front of each ear, and can be more easily located with mild palpation and, if necessary, requesting the patient to open their mouth slightly. The T3, C3, Cz, C4, and T4 electrodes are placed at marks made at intervals of 10%, 20%, 20%, 20%, 20%, and 10%, respectively, measured across the top of the head.
- Skull circumference is measured just above the ears (T3 and T4), just above the bridge of the nose (at Fpz), and just above the occipital point (at Oz). The Fp2, F8, T4, T6, and O2 electrodes are placed at intervals of 5%, 10%, 10%, 10%, 10%, and 5%, respectively, measured above the right ear, from front (Fpz) to back (Oz). The same is done for the odd-numbered electrodes on the left side, to complete the full circumference.
- Measurement methods for placement of the F3, F4, P3, and P4 points differ. If measured front-to-back (Fp1-F3-C3-P3-O1 and Fp2-F4-C4-P4-O2 montages), they can be 25% "up" from the front and back points (Fp1, Fp2, O1, and O2). If measured side to side (F7-F3-Fz-F4-F8 and T5-P3-Pz-P4-T6 montages), they can be 25% "up" from the side points (F7, F8, T5, and T6). If measured diagonally, from nasion to inion through the C3 and C4 points, they will be 20% in front of and behind the C3 and C4 points. Each of these measurement methods results in different nominal electrode placements.

When placing the A (or M) electrodes, palpation is often necessary to determine the most pronounced point of the mastoid process behind either ear; failure to do so, and to place the reference electrodes too low (posterior to the ear pinna, proximal to the throat) may result in "EKG artifact" in the EEGs and EOGs, due to artifact from the carotid arteries. EKG artifact can be reduced with post-filtering of signals, or by "jumping" (co-referencing) of A/M reference electrodes, if replacement of reference electrodes is not possible, ameliorative, or if other clinical considerations prevent otherwise good placement (such as congenital malformation, or post-surgical considerations such as cochlear implants) (Figure 5.4).

5.5 PLACEMENT OF THE EEG ELECTRODES FOR HIGHER-SPATIAL RESOLUTION

When recording a more detailed EEG with more electrodes, extra electrodes are added using *the 10% division*, which fills in intermediate sites halfway between those of the existing 10–20 system. This new electrode-naming-system is more complicated, giving rise to the modified combinatorial nomenclature (MCN). This MCN system uses 1, 3, 5, 7, 9 for the left hemisphere, which represents

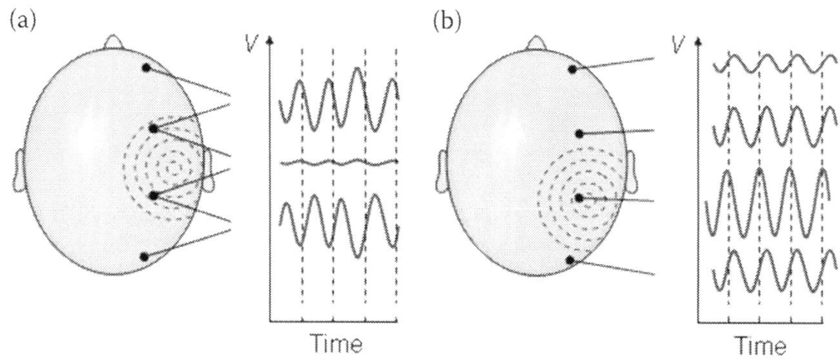

FIGURE 5.4 (a) Bipolar and (b) unipolar measurements. Note that the waveform of the EEG depends on the measurement location.

10%, 20%, 30%, 40%, and 50% of the inion-to-nasion distance, respectively. The introduction of extra letter codes allows the naming of intermediate electrode sites. Note that these new letter codes do not necessarily refer to an area on the underlying cerebral cortex. (Figure 5.5)

The new letter codes for indexing of the MCN for intermediate electrode places are:

- AF – between Fp and F
- FC – between F and C
- FT – between F and T
- CP – between C and P
- TP – between T and P
- PO – between P and O

Also, the MCN system renames four electrodes of the 10–20 system:

- T3 is now T7
- T4 is now T8
- T5 is now P7
- T6 is now P8

A higher-resolution nomenclature has been suggested and called the "5% system" or the "10–5 system."

5.5.1 Protocol for EEG Data Acquisition

EEG data acquisition is one of the vital steps of the entire chain of processing, inferring, and taking appropriate decision based on the behavior of EEG signal. Research analysts say "there is no substitute for clean data"; therefore, acquiring

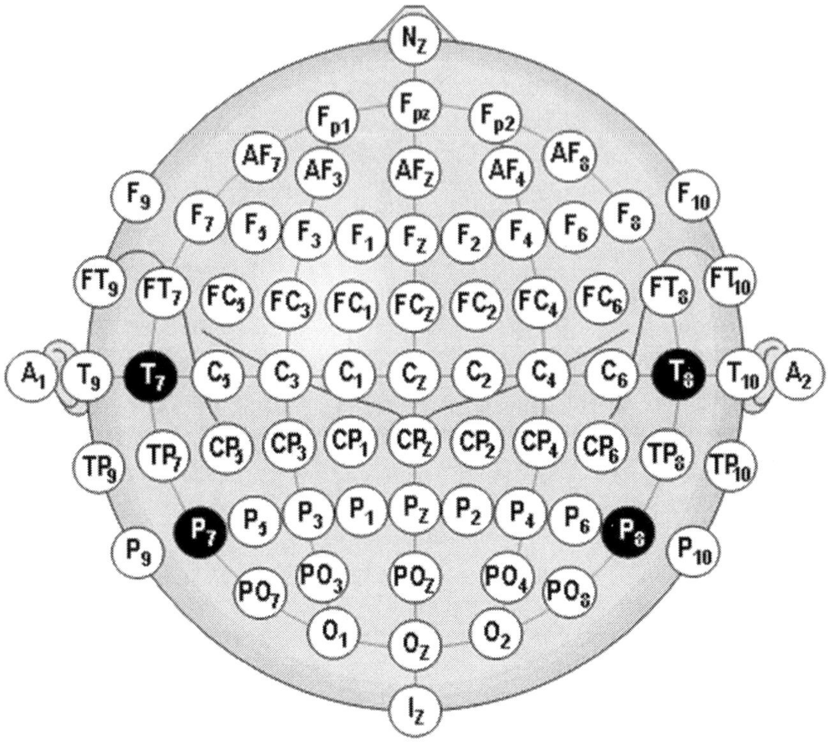

FIGURE 5.5 Location and nomenclature of the intermediate 10% electrodes, as standardized by the American Electroencephalographic Society.

clean EEG data devoid of noise is important. In order to acquire clean EEG data from a human subject, there are certain protocols followed both in the medical and research community. It is quite evident that the EEG is susceptible to noise as there are multiple sources of it. If proper measures are taken, then some of the noise sources can be prevented from affecting the signal of interest.

The resolution of the EEG data varies and it is dependent upon the number of electrodes in the EEG device and how the EEG probes are placed on the subjects' head for measurement. It can range from as low as 2 channels to as high as 256 channels (Figure 5.6). More channels give us a richer information and deeper insight into the activity of the brain. The electrodes used for recording can be varied based on the precision. As the raw EEG signal has a wide range of frequencies, the choice of frequency is also important. The frequency range of EEG is from 1 to 50 Hz. Thus, based on the application, the frequency needs to be filtered.

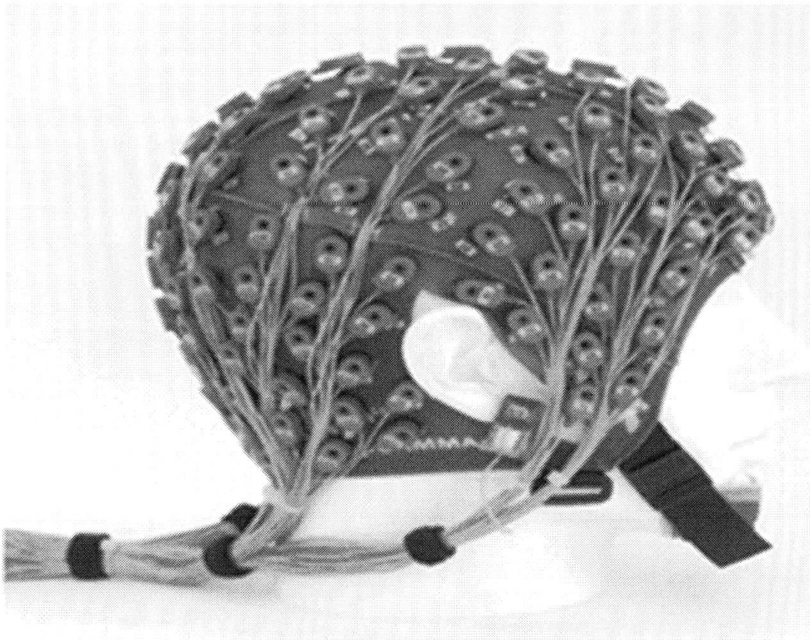

FIGURE 5.6 A 256-channel EEG cap.

5.5.2 Basic Protocol: Preparation of Human Subjects for EEG Acquisition

Before we advertise the experiment and gather participants, we have to decide on the subject criteria. Selected subjects have to meet all pre-determined requirements, that are designed to match the hypotheses, laws, and ethical regulations. The requirements that match the hypotheses differ from experiment to experiment. The requirements that match laws and regulations are common for all EEG experiments. This ensures the safety of all participants.

Common criteria for selection of the subject for EEG acquisition:

- General good health
- No pregnancy
- No claustrophobia
- No drug addiction
- No neurological diseases

Specific selection criteria that differs from experiment to experiment to take into account:

- Range of age
- One or both genders

- Academic level
- Specific type of disease or the absence of it (in case of studies on dementia or other diseases)
- Visual acuity and/or hearing acuity (depending on the type of stimuli which subjects are exposed to during the experiment)
- If the person is left handed or right handed

5.5.3 Subjects' Data Selection

Often the data acquired from a subject is clear enough to process it for further investigation. Therefore, the data can be rejected. Some of the reasons to reject the recorded data of a subject are:

- Lack of signal for a specific time window
- External sudden electrical noises that interfere and ruin the signal
- Electrodes shifting or falling due to discomfort of the subject that cause the signal to drop
- Improper gelling of the contact between the scalp and the electrodes

It is recommended to check the data before starting the processing. In the case of missing data, the subject can be rejected or brought in again for additional tests or minor adjustments can be made to restore proper collection of the data.

5.5.4 EEG Acquisition Setup Block

Figure 5.7 shows the general block for acquiring the signal during an experiment using visual or auditory evoked potentials.

The amplifier amplifies the signal to ensure the signal is in the range of uV readable to the user and it also performs frequency filtering if asked.

- The stimulus presenter is used to show the presentation of the task the user is given. The response box is a set of keys that the user can press if the task requires the subject to do so.
- A camera is used to record the subject's behavior and, if possible, to perform the eye tracking if required.

5.5.5 Experimental Procedure

5.5.5.1 Recruiting Subjects

- Advertise the experiments and the subjects' requirements within fellow research groups, hospitals, and medical centers.
- Screen possible choices and arrange appointment for testing.
- Instruct the subject to come to the test with just washed hair and no hair products, and to be on their best physical and mental conditions.

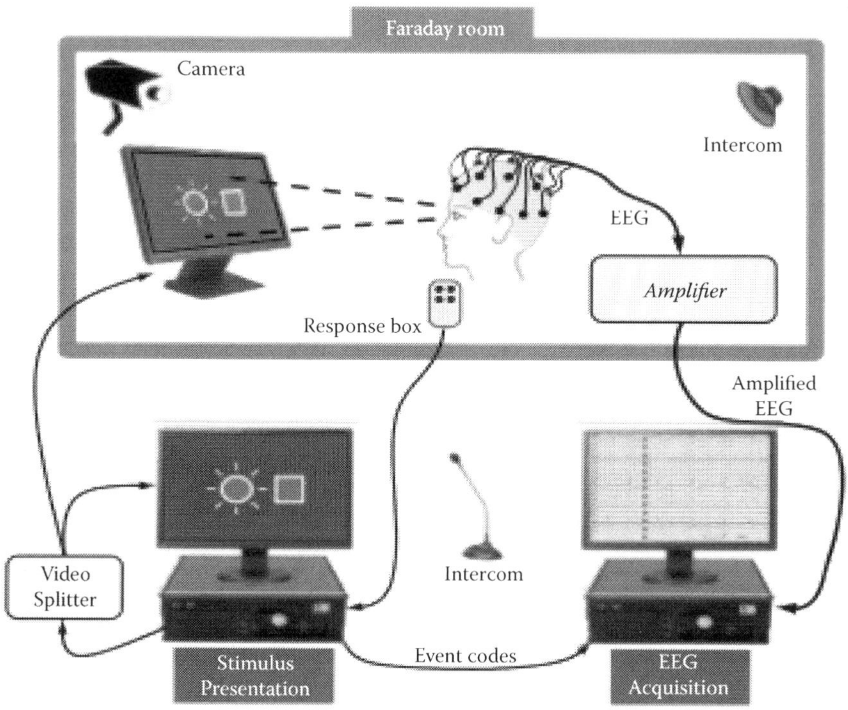

FIGURE 5.7 Schematics of an EEG acquisition setup.

5.5.5.2 Before the Experiment

- Prepare information notice, instruction paper, and consent paper
- Verify and test the setup, the stimulation system and routine, and the hardware in the workspace
- Check connection with recording system
- Prepare your gel syringes if you are using wet electrodes

5.5.5.3 During the Experiment

- Welcome the subject into the lab and make them feel comfortable
- Explain the experiment and make sure the subject is clear on any aspect of it
- Have subject sign the consent paper
- Adjust the stimulation setup to the subject's comfort (adjust chair height, screen distance, or check sound)
- Prepare head and secure selected cap
- Perform impedance measurement
- Perform testing
- Verify the obtained signal is properly electrophysiological
- Keep the subject attentive and motivated; allow for breaks

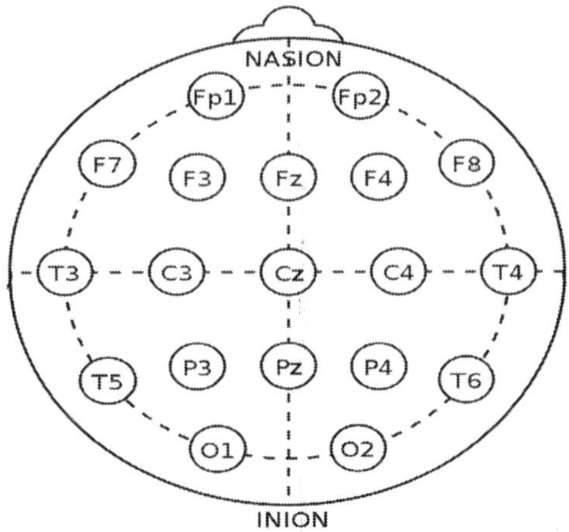

FIGURE 5.8 Cross-sectional view of 10–20 electrode placement diagram.

In our experiment, Axxonet's Brain Electro Scan System (BESS), which is a 32-channel EEG system, was used to record the EEG data of the subjects. The system has a maximum sampling rate per channel of 30 kbps and runs on 5 V AC supply. Gold-plated silver electrodes soaked in saline water were used. The detection of beta waves (16–31 Hz), which are responsible for cognitive actions like thinking, planning, focusing, high alert etc., are profoundly observed over the recorded data. Initially, a notch filter of 0.5 to 75 Hz was applied. T8, CP6, A1, and A2 channels were used to record EOG data and 10–20 electrode placement system was used to record the EEG data. Depicted in Figure 5.8 is the cross-sectional view of the electrode placement to capture the EEG.

5.6 EOG DATA ACQUISITION

Before starting the recording session for acquisition of the EEG, the subject was asked to stay as calm as possible during the test (see Figure 6.3 in Chapter 6). First, a scene containing the picture of an object was shown to the subject, followed by a different scene containing several instances of the same object in different locations in the scenes. The subject was instructed to read the scene and identify the objects in the scene. During this process, the EEG of the subject is acquired and recorded. This experiment can be conducted on different subjects and for the same scene.

While recording the EEG, the distance from the monitor to the subject is kept at a distance of 93 cm. The monitor size is (30 × 60 cm^2). The distance from the camera to the subject is 27 cm. The camera feed is used for gaze estimation and provide approximate coordinates of the eye-fix on the monitor screen.

5.7 SUMMARY

EEG acquisition is a vital step in the process of the entire experiment. The isolation of the noise is of high priority in order to get a pure EEG signal. In this way, one would be required to employ noise removal techniques in the first place. Subject selection and subject awareness play the most important role while performing this experiment. Without proper precautionary measures, there is every possibility of the signal being corrupted and mixed with noise.

Exercises

1. What is the standard topology for placement of electrodes on the scalp? Discuss the international standard followed.
2. Discuss the alternate electrode placement and indexing method adopted for placement of electrodes for normal EEG data acquisition and for high-resolution data acquisition.
3. What are unipolar and bipolar EEG data accquisition?
4. What are 10–20, 10–10, and 10–5 electrode placement systems?
5. What are the common criteria for selection of the subject for EEG accquisition?
6. List some of the specific criteria for selecting subjects for EEG acquisition.
7. Give a generic protocol followed before EEG acquisition.
8. Present a block diagram describing the entire process of EEG acquisition.
9. Describe the EEG acquisition setup through a schematic diagram.
10. Draw a cross-sectional view of a 10–20 electrode placement and describe its significance.

REFERENCES

Berger, H 1929, 'Über das Elektroenkephalogramm des Menschen.' *Arch Psychiatr Nervenkr*, vol. 87, pp. 527–570.

Blumhardt, LD, Barrett, G, Halliday, AM & Kriss, A 1977, 'The asymmetrical visual evoked potential to pattern reversal in one half field and its significance for the analysis of visual field effects,' *British Journal of Ophthalmology*, vol. 61, pp. 454–461.

Chatrian, GE, Lettich, E & Nelson, PL 1985, 'Ten percent electrode system for topographic studies of spontaneous and evoked EEG activity.' *American Journal of Electroneurodiagnostic Technology*, vol. 25, pp. 83–92.

Clerc, M, Bougrain, L & Lotte, F (eds.) 2016 August 30, *Brain–Computer Interfaces: Technology and Applications*, doi:10.1002/9781119332428

Cooper, R, Osselton, JW & Shaw, JC 1969, *EEG Technology*, 2nd ed., pp. 275. Butterworths, London.

Electrode Position Nomenclature Committee 1991 April, 'American electroencephalographic society guidelines for standard electrode position nomenclature' *Journal of Clinical Neurophysiology*, vol. 8, no. 2, pp. 200–202. doi:10.1097/00004691-1991 04000-00007. PMID 2050819. S2CID 11857141.

Electrode Position Nomenclature Committee, *Journal of Clinical Neurophysiology* 1994 January, 'Guideline thirteen,' vol. 11, no. 1, pp. 111–113. doi:10.1097/00004691-199401000-00014. PMID 8195414.

Gilmore, RL 1994 January, 'American Electroencephalographic Society guidelines in electroencephalography, evoked potentials, and polysomnography,' *Journal of Clinical Neurophysiology*, vol. 11, no.1, p. 147.

Jasper, HH 1958 May, 'Report of the committee on methods of clinical examination in electroencephalography,' *Electroencephalography and Clinical Neurophysiology*, vol. 10, no. 2, pp. 370–375. doi:10.1016/0013-4694(58)90053-1

Klem, GH, Lüders, HO, Jasper, HH & Elger, C 1999, 'The ten-twenty electrode system of he International Federation. The International Federation of Clinical Neurophysiology,' *Electroencephalography and Clinical Neurophysiology. Supplement*, vol. 52, pp. 3–6. PMID 10590970.

Niedermeyer, E & da Silva FL 2004, *Electroencephalography: Basic Principles, Clinical Applications, and Related Fields*, pp. 140, Lippincott Williams & Wilkins, New York. ISBN 0-7817-5126-8, ISBN 978-0-7817-5126-1.

Nunez, PL 1981, *Electric Fields of the Brain: The Neurophysics of EEG*, pp. 484, Oxford University Press, New York.

Nuwer, MR, Comi, G, Emerson, R, Fuglsang-Frederiksen, A, Guérit, J-M, Hinrichs, H, Ikeda, A, Luccas, FJ & Rappelsburger, P 1998 March, 'IFCN standards for digital recording of clinical EEG,' *Electroencephalography and Clinical Neurophysiology*, vol. 106, no. 3, pp. 259–261. doi:10.1016/S0013-4694(97)001 06-5. PMID 9743285.

Oostenveld, R & Praamstra, P 2001, 'The five percent electrode system for high-resolution EEG and ERP measurements,' *Clinical Neurophysiology*, vol. 112, no. 4, pp. 713–719. CiteSeerX 10.1.1.116.7379. doi:10.1016/S1388-2457(00)00527-7. PMID 11275545. S2CID 15414860.

Puikkonen, J & Malmivuo, JA 1987, 'Theoretical investigation of the sensitivity distribution of point EEG-electrodes on the three concentric spheres model of a human head – An application of the reciprocity theorem,' *Tampere University of Technology, Institute of Biomedical Engineering, Reports*, vol. 1, no. 5, p. 71.

Rush, S & Driscoll, DA 1969, 'EEG-electrode sensitivity - An application of reciprocity,' *IEEE Transactions on Biomedical Engineering*, vol. BME-16, no. 1, pp. 15–22.

Sharbrough, F, Chatrian, G-E, Lesser, RP, Lüders, H, Nuwer, M & Picton, TW 1991, 'American electroencephalographic society guidelines for standard electrode position nomenclature,' *Journal of Clinical Neurophysiology*, vol. 8, pp. 200–202.

Suihko, V, Malmivuo, JA & Eskola, H 1993, 'Distribution of sensitivity of electric leads in an inhomogeneous spherical head model,' *Tampere University of Technology, Ragnar Granit Institute*, Report, vol. 7, no. 2.

6 Methods to Detect Blink from the EEG Signal

OVERVIEW

This chapter discusses the method to detect the blink artifacts from the EEG signal. It discusses the applications and use of the presence of blinks in the EEG data. The process of acquisition of EOG data and its algorithm to process and extract blinks from EOG are explained. The algorithm is applied on the data acquired from different subjects and the output is discussed.

6.1 INTRODUCTION

An electroencephalogram (EEG) is a measure of the electrical signals of the brain of a human being. It is a readily available test that provides the evidence of how the brain functions over time. Brain computer interface (BCI) is a collaboration between a brain and a device that enables EEG signals from the brain to control some external activity, such as control of a cursor or a prosthetic limb (Roy et al 2011). The interface enables a direct communication pathway between the brain and the object to be controlled. Electrooculography (EOG) is a technique for measuring the corneo-retinal standing potential that exists between the front and the back of the human eye. The resulting signal is called the electrooculogram. Tracking the movement of the eye through sensors enables us to compute and fix the position where one's eyes are focused (Panigrahi et al 2019). Study of the EOG can determine presence, attention, focus, drowsiness, consciousness, or other mental states of the subject (TejeroGimeno et al 2006; Liu et al 2013; Lin et al 2005). Event related potential (ERP) is a small voltage generated in the brain due to the occurrence of a specific event or stimuli. ERPs can be reliably measured from an EEG.

In this research, we characterize the EEG signal and propose a method to detect and process the EOG signal. When active, i.e., not in the state of sleep, the external functioning of human eye is characterized by three distinct functions: saccadic, fix, and blink. Saccadic and fix are voluntary actions or actions controlled by humans, whereas the blink is an involuntary action that is associated with randomness and high fluctuation of EEG voltage (Landau et al 2007). We discuss how to capture the EEG and EOG signals and how to filter the EEG channel to delineate the EOG and related signals from other channels. Then we discuss the process to characterize and delineate the blinks from the rest of the EEG signals so that saccadic and fix are delineated.

DOI: 10.1201/9781003241386-6

6.2 PROCESS OF EEG DATA ACQUISITION

In our experiment, Axxonet's Brain Electro Scan System (BESS), which is a 32-channel EEG system, was used to record the EEG data of the subjects. The system has a maximum sampling rate per channel of 30 kps and runs on 5 V AC supply. Gold-plated silver electrodes soaked in saline water were used. The detection of beta waves (16–31 Hz), which are responsible for cognitive actions like thinking, planning, focusing, high alert etc., are profoundly observed over the recorded data. Initially, a notch filter of 0.5 to 75 Hz was applied. T8, CP6, A1, and A2 channels were used to record EOG data. The 10–20 electrode placement system is used to record EEG data. Depicted in Figure 6.1 and Figure 6.2 is the cross-sectional view of the electrode placement to capture the EEG and one of the subject while capturing the EEG data, respectively.

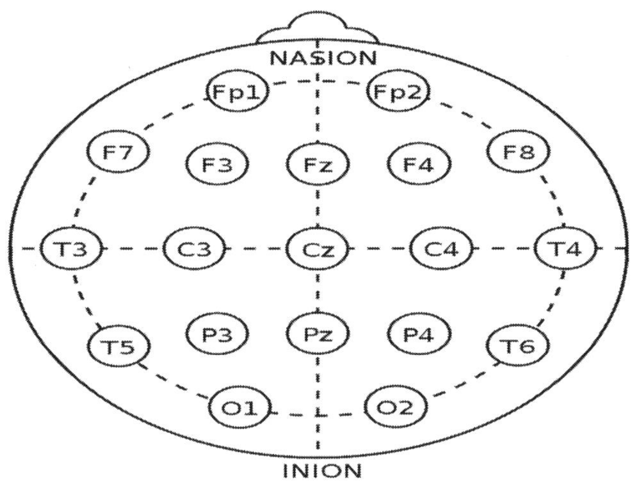

FIGURE 6.1 Cross sectional view of 10-20 electrode placement diagram.

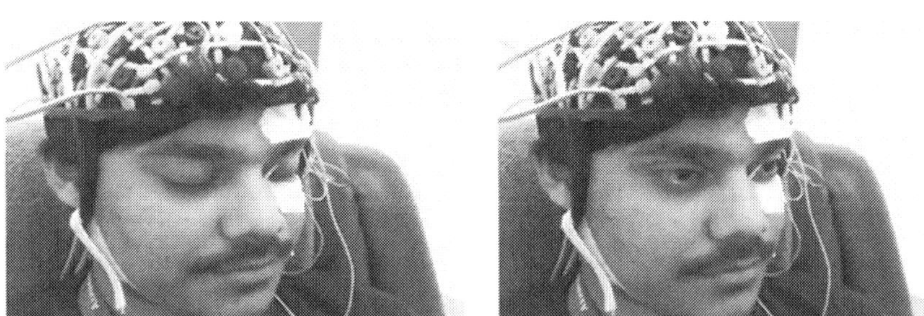

FIGURE 6.2 EOG electrode placement on subject. (Courtesy Axxonet Pvt. Ltd., Bangalore, India.)

6.3 EOG DATA ACQUISITION

Before starting the recording session for acquisition of the EEG, the subject was asked to stay as calm as possible during the test. First, a scene containing the picture of an object was shown to the user. Then, five slides containing several instances of the object in different locations of the scene were displayed. The subject was instructed to read the scene and identify the objects in the scenc. During this process, the EEG of the subject was acquired and recorded. This experiment was conducted on different subjects and on the same scene. The process is depicted in Figure 6.3. The EEG acquired from the subject is plotted in Figure 6.4.

While recording EEG, the distance from monitor to the subject is kept at a distance of 93 cm. The monitor size is (30 × 60 cm^2). The distance from the camera to the subject is 27 cm. The camera feed is used for gaze estimation and it provides approximate coordinates of the eye-fix on the monitor screen.

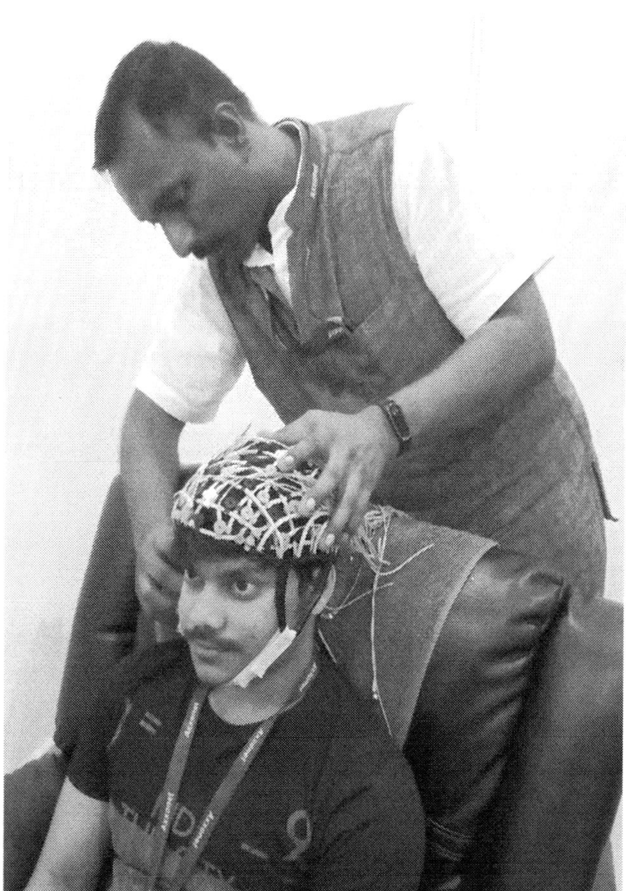

FIGURE 6.3 Subject wearing EEG cap while recording of EEG and EOG signal. (Courtesy Axxonet Pvt. Ltd., Bangalore, India.)

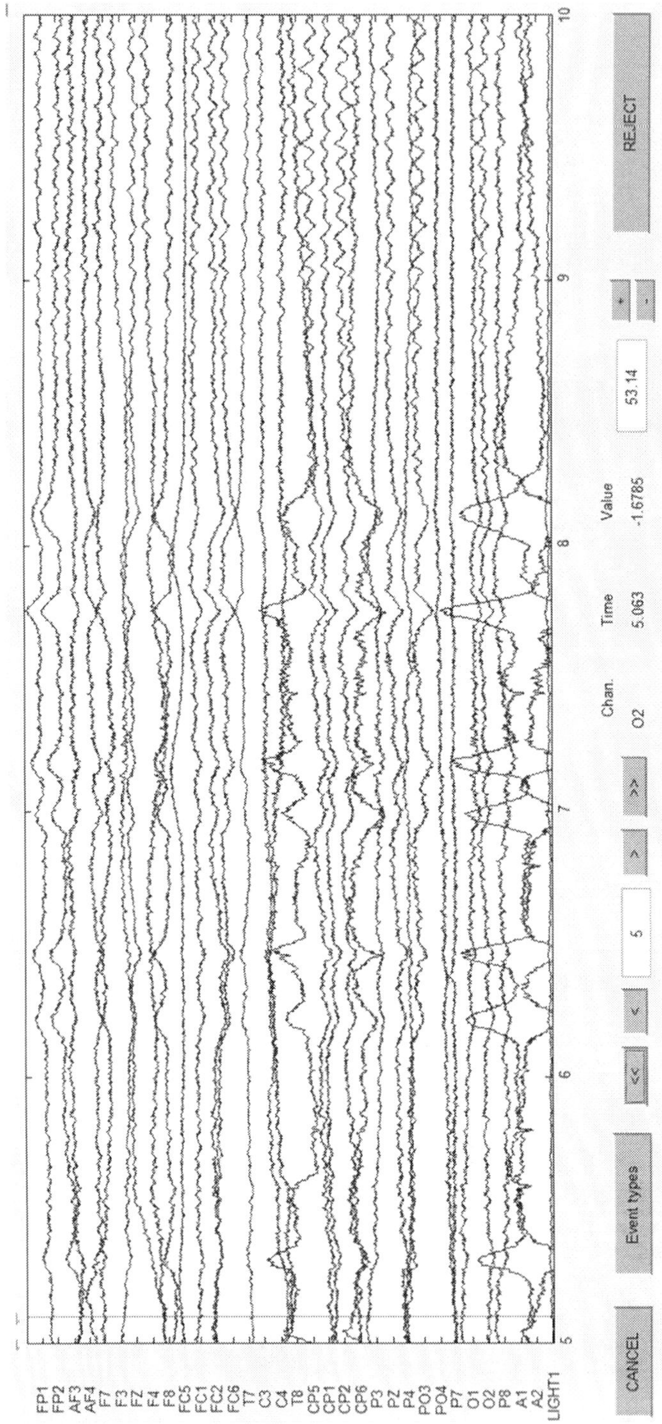

FIGURE 6.4 32 Channel EEG data plot using EEGLAB Toolbox (Version 14.1.2b).

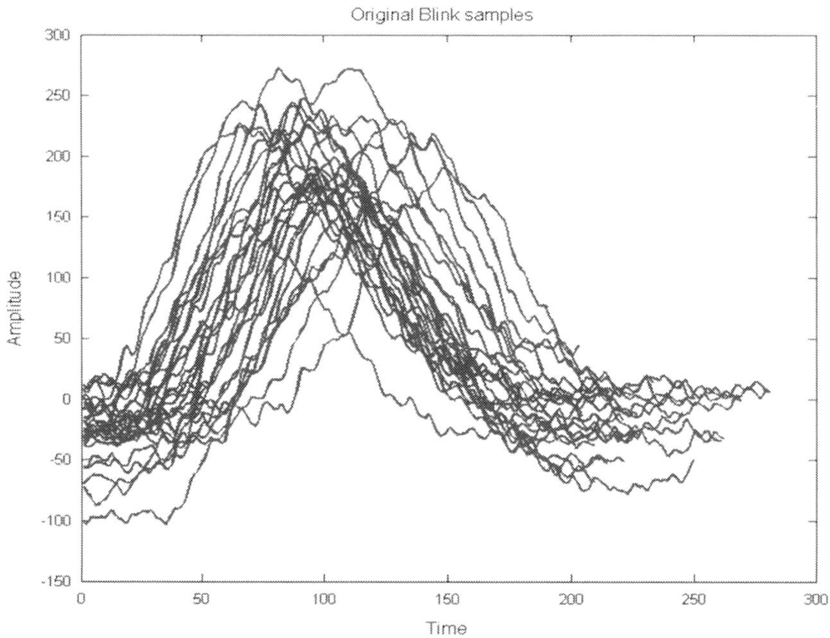

FIGURE 6.5 Overlapped Plot of 29 blink samples.

6.4 BLINK DETECTION

The EEG signal has the characteristic that it has highly varying in voltage and frequency. Also, the baseband of the signal varies frequently in time. Therefore, the EEG truly represents the variation of mind in space and time.

Blinks in EEG and EOG signals are considered artifacts in the EEG. To filter and detect the blink from the EEG, we propose a novel technique of blink detection.

Step 1. EEG data acquired in .edf format is loaded in MATLAB® using the EEGLAB toolbox (version 14.1.2b).

Step 2. Plot the EEG acquired in step 1 to visualize the recorded data for all channels. Sampling rate was set to 1,024 Hz.

Step 3. The application was mostly concerned with frequencies in the range of 0–30 Hz. We filtered the overall channel signals into 1–30 Hz frequency using a standard filtering technique available in the EEGLAB toolbox. After visual analysis of the plot obtained, it is found that the impact of the blinks was mostly affecting the signal obtained from FP1, FP2, A1(EOG1), and A2(EOG2). Hence, the signal obtained from these four channels was used for further processing of blink artifact.

Step 4. After filtering, the signal contained too many fluctuations over a very short time period. In order to get rid of unwanted fluctuations and make the signals smoother, the signals were subjected to a moving average technique. Figure 6.5 illustrates the results obtained for two individual blink occurrences.

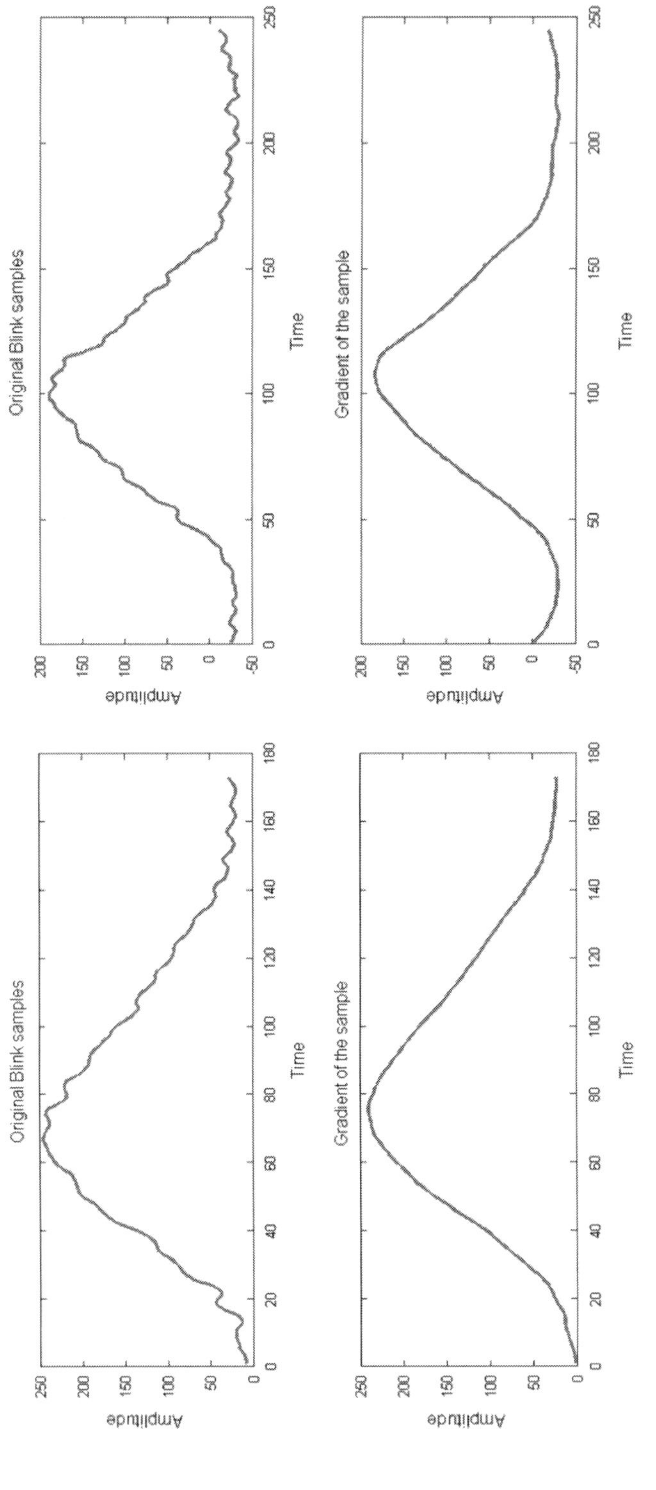

FIGURE 6.6 Two blink samples and the resulting signal after applying Moving Average technique.

As shown in Figure 6.6, the DC value for each individual blink sample is highly variant; therefore, the standard threshold technique will produce very poor results if applied. Thus, calculation of the gradient for the signal will result in better detection of the activity of the peaks caused by blinks.

Step 5. Blinks were detected using the following method:

- The signal from channel EOG1 was selected and the moving average technique was applied on it with a lead parameter value 10 and lag parameter value 20. The result is shown in Figure 6.7, first subplot.
- The gradient of the signal was obtained and shown in the second subplot.

Step 6. A modified threshold technique was applied on the gradient to obtain the duration of each individual blink. The threshold function is defined as below:

$$f(x) = \begin{cases} 2T, & x \geq T \\ T, & 0 \leq x < T \\ -T, & 0 > x > -T \\ -2T, & x \geq -T \end{cases}$$

Where,

$$T = C * argmax(|x|)$$
$$C = 0.3$$

C is a constant that needs to be adjusted for proper blink detection, generally in the range (0.1 to 0.5).

Step 7. After applying the threshold function, in the resultant starting and ending points of the blink are highlighted on the original signal and shown in the fourth subplot. Hence, this technique of blink detection was applied on the whole signal and for all selected channels.

6.5 RESULTS

The algorithm was tested on two subjects' recordings and the corresponding results are shown in Table 6.1.

Due to the lengthy size of the data, we divided the data into a range of 30,000 data points (29.3 s as sampling rate is 1,024 Hz) and analyzed them one by one. The constant C was adjusted for each data point range, but it was observed to be the same throughout the course of the experiment. Similarly, the lag and the lead for the moving average applied on the signal was also found to be same. These parameters were found to be the best for detection. Too high values of lead and lag led to omission of the blinks and too low values of the lead and lag led to noisy blink signatures.

Taking the data of subject 1 into consideration, it was observed that subject 1 blinked frequently during the course of the experiment. A total of 130 blinks were recorded manually, out of which 85 were correctly detected, which gives an accuracy of 65%. The subject was tired while performing this experiment with

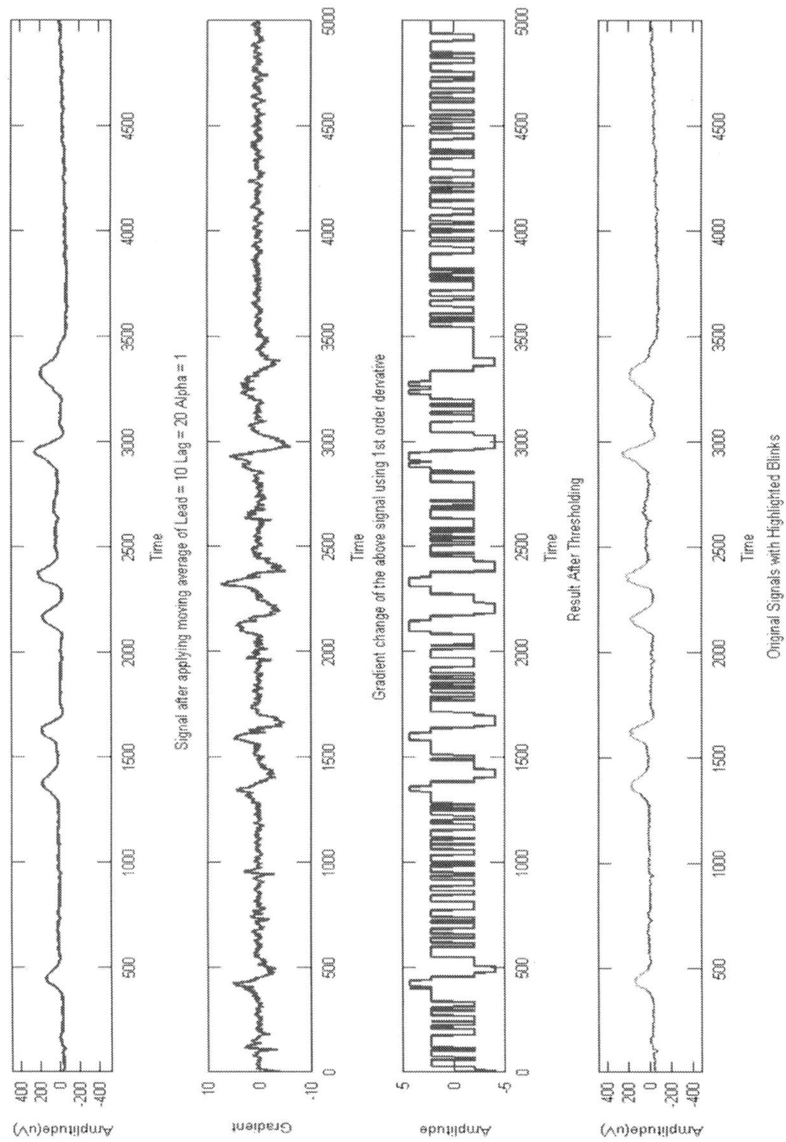

FIGURE 6.7 Detection of blinks in EEG data stream.

TABLE 6.1
Algorithm accuracy verified for EEG data obtained from two subjects

Subject	Data Point Range (x1000)	C	Lag	Lead	No of Blinks Present	True Positives	False Negatives	Accuracy (%)
1	5-30	0.3	5	10	11	8	0	65.38
	30-60	0.3	5	10	14	8	0	
	60-90	0.3	5	10	31	19	1	
	90-120	0.3	5	10	25	14	1	
	120-160	0.3	5	10	27	23	2	
	160-180	0.3	5	10	13	9	0	
	180-198.656	0.3	5	10	9	4	2	
2	5-35	0.2	5	10	6	5	1	90
	35-65	0.3	5	10	1	1	0	
	65-95	0.3	5	10	1	1	0	
	95-125	0.3	5	10	-	-	-	
	125-185	0.3	5	10	1	1	0	
	185-204.8	0.3	5	10	1	1	0	

signs of drowsiness. Consecutively, such a high blink rate was observed as it was difficult to concentrate on the task.

On the other hand, subject 2 was well rested and relaxed throughout the experiment a total of ten blinks were recorded manually out of which nine were detected successfully. Thus, the detection accuracy was 90%. Subjects 1 and 2 were given the same set of tasks to perform. As subject 2 was well rested, it can be concluded easily that the subject performed the task with a very low blink rate as the concentration level was high.

6.6 APPLICATIONS

Applications of blink detection are many (the source code for detection of blink artifact is listed in the Appendix). One of them is the determination of one's concentration level and drowsiness. It was found according to the latest research (Bentivoglio et al 1997) that the mean blink rate at rest was 17 blinks per minute and during conversation it increased to 26 and it was as low as 4.5 while reading. Based on the statistics, we can infer that a subject's concentration level is high if they have a blink rate of at most 6 per minute. Otherwise, the subject is either low in their concentration level or distracted. However, if it is observed that the blink duration of the subject is above a certain level, then the subject is feeling drowsy. Blink is considered an artifact during EEG analysis. Therefore, detection of blinks is used to remove them from the original signal for further analysis.

6.7 SUMMARY

The methodology used in the experiment includes gradient calculation and a modified threshold function to detect the blinks in EEG signals. As a result, this method for detecting blinks is computationally cost effective compared to other traditional methods (Sawant & Jalali 2010, HafeezUllah et al 2017, Lotte et al 2007). Blinks can also be used to measure alertness, drowsiness, and other cognitive states. In the future research can be extended towards future research can be extended towards detection of different mind states by using the blink detection technique. Further pattern recognition techniques using deep neural networks with a multiclass classifier can be implemented to recognize cognitive states.

Exercises

1. What is EOG and how do you acquire EOG data?
2. What is a blink and which part of the brain or neural segment regulates a blink?
3. What is the use of a blink and which psychological and philological states of a human can be detected from a blink?
4. Discuss the step-wise processing to extract blinks from EOG signals.
5. Discuss the modified threshold technique to extract blinks from an EEG.

REFERENCES

Bentivoglio AR, Bressman SB, Cassetta E, Carretta D, Tonali P & Albanese A 1997 November, 'Analysis of blink rate patterns in normal subjects,' *IEEE Potential*, vol. 12, no. 6, pp. 1028–1034. DOI:10.1002/mds.870120629.

HafeezUllah, A, Wajid, M, Rauf, SA, Mohamad, SMN & Saeed, MA 2017, 'Classification of EEG signals based on pattern recognition approach,' *Frontiers in Computational Neuroscience*, vol. 11, pp. 1662–5188. doi:10.3389/fncom.2017.00103.

Landau, AN, Esterman, M, Robertson, LC, Bentin, S & Prinzmetal, W 2007, 'Different effects of voluntary and involuntary attention on EEG activity in the gamma band,' *The Journal of Neuroscience*, vol. 27, no. 44, pp. 11986–11990.

Lin, C-T, et al. 2005, 'EEG-based drowsiness estimation for safety driving using independent component analysis,' *IEEE Transactions on Circuits and Systems I: Regular Papers*, vol. 52, no. 12, pp. 2726–2738.

Liu, N-H, Chiang, C-Y & Chu, H-C 2013, 'Recognizing the degree of human attention using EEG signals from mobile sensors,' *Sensors*, vol. 13, pp. 10273–10286. doi: 10.3390/s130810273.

Lotte, F, et al. 2007, 'A review of classification algorithms for EEG-based brain–computer interfaces,' *Journal of Neural Engineering*, vol. 4, no. 2, p. R1. doi:10.1088/1741-2560/4/2/R01.

Panigrahi, N, Lavu, K, Gorijala, SK, Corcoran, P & Mohanty, SP 2019 January–February, 'A method for localizing the eye pupil for point-of-gaze estimation,' in *IEEE Potentials*, vol. 38, no. 1, pp. 37–42. doi:10.1109/MPOT.2018.2850540 keywords: {Eyes;Gazetracking;Videos;Digital images}, URL: http://ieeexplore.ieee.org/stamp/stamp.jsp?tp=&arnumber=8595416&isnumber=8595411

Roy, R, Konar, A & Tibarewala, DN 2011, 'Control of artificial limb using EEG and EMG – A review,' in *AICTE Sponsored National Conference, BERA-2011*, JIS College of Engineering, India, July 2011.

Sawant, HK & Jalali, Z 2010, 'Detection and classification of EEG waves,' *Oriental Journal of Computer Science and Technology*, vol. 3, no. 1, pp. 207–213.

Tejero Gimeno, P, Pastor, G & Choliz, M 2006, 'On the concept and measurement of driver drowsiness, fatigue and inattention: Implications for countermeasures,' *International Journal of Vehicle Design*, vol. 42, pp. 67–86. doi:10.1504/IJVD.2006.010178.

7 Saccade and Fix Detection from EOG Signals

OVERVIEW

This chapter discusses different methods employed to detect and segregate the saccade and fixation from the EOG data. The entire process of saccade and fixation detection from EOG data is elucidated through a block diagram. The varying baseline of the EEG data is characterized. A baseline drift removal algorithm is proposed and discussed in this chapter.

7.1 INTRODUCTION

The physical activities of human eye constitute of three repetitive activities: saccade, fix, and blink. Blinking is an involuntary action; the saccades and fix correspond to different cognitive actions of human beings (Panigrahi et al 2019a). Often these actions are guided with active correlation of actions of neurological activities of the brain. A saccade is defined by the movement of the eyeball from one viewpoint to another. A saccade action can be captured through the EOG signal that is characterized by sudden deflection of the voltage fluctuation in the EOG. Study and analysis of saccadic movement and its pattern has many applications that can lead to the understanding of cognitive capabilities of human beings (Panigrahi et al. 2019b).

The advancement of an EEG acquisition system and development of sophisticated computing methods to process EOG signals has led to its widespread applications. Artifacts of EEG signals are being used to control IoT devices, to compute cognitive capabilities and agility of the mind, to forecast any epileptic activity, etc.

Here, we propose a method to compute and delineate the EEG signal. We apply a wavelet decomposition transform followed by a median filter to segregate the EEG signal corresponding to the saccadic movement. In this process, first we apply the wavelet denoising transform (Patil & Chavan 2012) to remove the local fluctuations from the signal. Then, CWT is applied to find the coefficients required to detect the saccades and eventually the fixes.

Finally, we design a function that uses positive and negative thresholds to detect the saccadic movements in the signal. It is observed that fixations are interleaved by way of two saccades of the eye (Henderson & Andrew 2003;

DOI: 10.1201/9781003241386-7

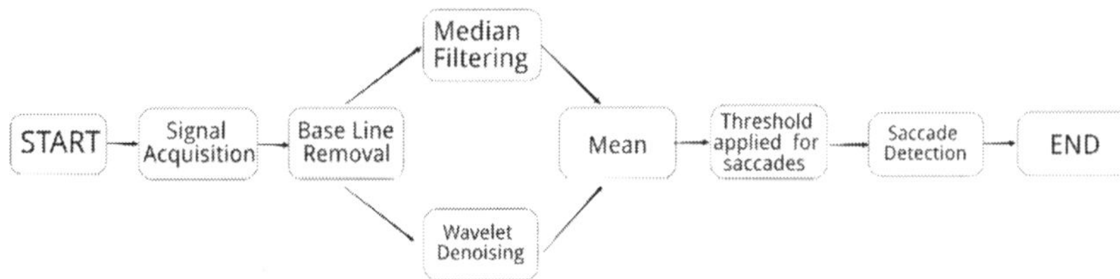

FIGURE 7.1 Block diagram for Saccade detection system.

Henn & Cohen 1973). This process of saccade detection in the EOG signal is performed after removing the baseline DC value. This process is depicted in the block diagram given in Figure 7.1.

7.2 METHODS

7.2.1 Block Diagram

The overall block diagram depicting the process of delineating saccade and fixation from EOG data is given in Figure 7.1. The process uses the baseline removal algorithm, which is a new technique implemented and experimented. The result of the baseline-removed EEG signal along with the original signal is plotted in Figure 7.2 for comparison. The two distinct approaches experimented to detect the saccade from the EEG signal are

a. EEG Signal → Baseline Removal → Median Filtering → Thresholding of Signal for Saccade → Saccade Detection
b. EEG Signal → Base ine Removal → Wavelet Denoising → Thresholding for Saccade → Saccade Detection

7.2.2 Baseline Drift Removal

Baseline drift is the short time variation of the baseline from a straight line caused by electric signal fluctuations. Baseline drift can occur due to breathing, loose contact between electrode and skin, or body movement. It compromises the information content in the signal. In order to remove this, we performed multilevel 1D wavelet decomposition at level 12 using a reverse bi-orthogonal wavelet "rbio6.8" (Gupta & Singh 1996). Reverse bi-orthogonal wavelets are obtained by bi-orthogonal wavelet pairs that exhibit linear properties that are advantageous for our experiment.

Figure 7.2 represents the comparison between the original signal and signal after baseline drift removal. Baseline drift removal results in proper analysis of the signal as described above. As discussed in Chapter 3, the sources of baseline wander maybe different, but it always appears as a low-frequency artifact that introduces slow oscillations in the recorded signal.

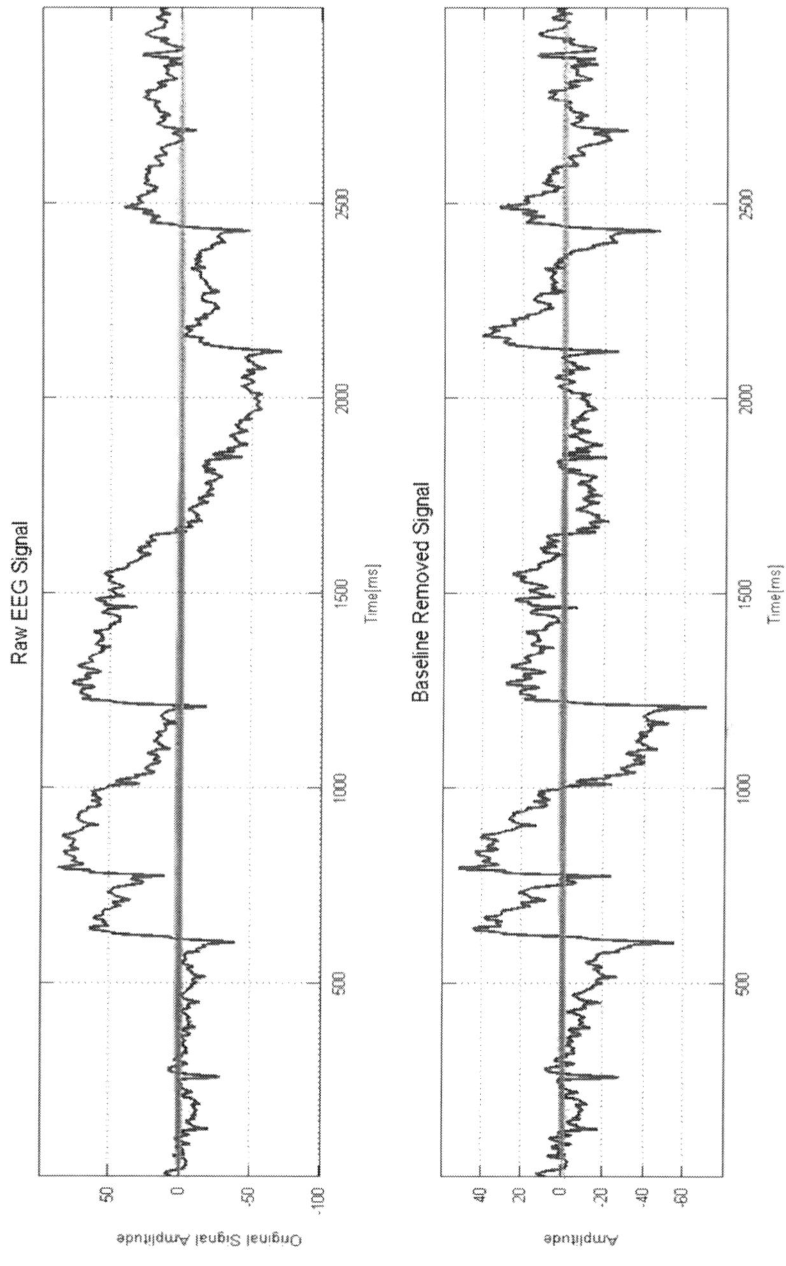

FIGURE 7.2 Comparison of the original signal and baseline-removed signal.

7.2.3 Noise Removal

We observed that the information contained in the EOG signal had noise, which affected the process of detection of the saccades. This was due to bad placement of the electrodes, muscle twitches, random head movements, and local electrical interferences. The removal of this noise required careful selection of the filtering technique to be applied. Based on our research, median filtering and wavelet denoising appeared to be best suited for our problem.

7.2.4 Median Filtering

Median filtering is a window-based noise removal technique where the window takes the median of its values and replaces them with it. For our problem, it was particularly helpful as it preserved the steep nature of the saccades. However, the window size of the median filter was a matter of concern as large windows distorted the edge and shape of the saccades and also possibly removed the small saccades. As a result, it was a trade-off between precision versus noise.

For our application, the order of the filter was varied between 10 and 40 and it was visually observed and concluded that the best possible parameter was a median filter of 19 order and window size of 74 ms. This filter not only prevented the removal of small saccades of interests but also successfully removed the noise that was present. Figure 7.3 describes the comparison of the process.

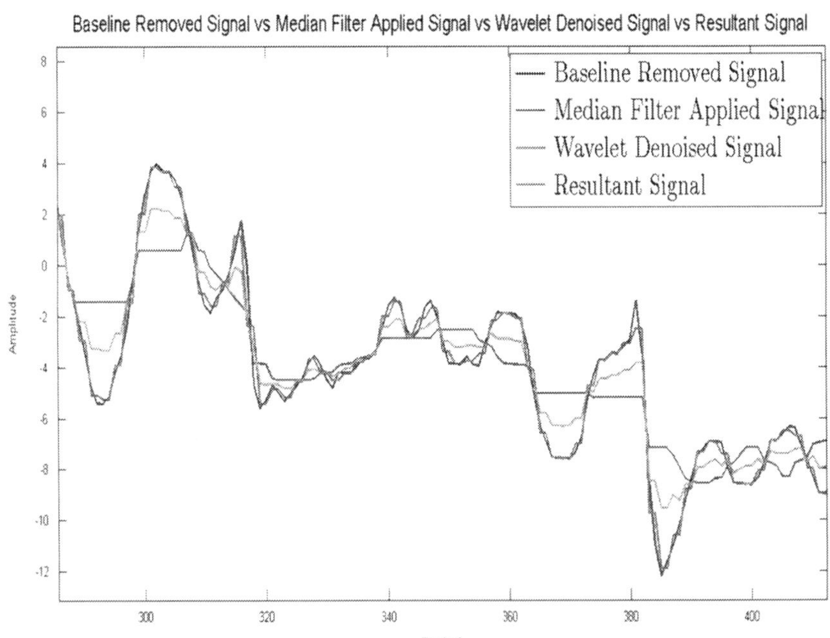

FIGURE 7.3 Illustration of filtering techniques applied on the signal.

7.2.5 Wavelet Denoising

Wavelet denoising is a noise removal technique where the mother wavelet is passed through the signal and the correlation coefficients are obtained (Gao et al 2010). After that, a soft/hard thresholding is applied that removes the low amplitude noise from the signal.

For our application, the built-in MATLAB® function "wden" was used to perform the denoising. The signal was denoised using the "Symlet" wavelet of level 1 and soft thresholding was applied on the coefficients with a universal threshold th = $\sqrt{lnlnN}$, where N is the length of the time series.

The results of the noise removal obtained independently were taken and were averaged out and the resulting signal obtained was devoid of noise of higher frequency.

7.2.6 Saccade Detection

Saccades are observed as abrupt changes in voltage (similar to step functions). Continuous wavelet transform (CWT) (Du et al 2006; Nenadic & Burdick 2005) is very sensitive to this kind of change. We applied the "Haar" mother wavelet with a scale of 20 at level 12 to the signal after baseline removal and denoising (Bulling et al 2011). The Haar wavelet is a sequence of rescaled "square-shaped" functions that together form a wavelet. Therefore, due to similarity with the saccade's shape, the Haar wavelet was chosen to carry on the experiment.

A threshold of ±25 was applied on the resulting CWT coefficients. Positive and negative peaks above the thresholds were marked to represent the occurrence of the saccades. Corresponding points were also marked in the original signal and the result is given in Figure 7.4.

7.2.7 Fixation

A subject maintaining constant visual gaze on any particular location is known as fixation. The term "fixation" can either be used to refer to the point in time and space of focus or the act of fixating. Gaze points show what the eyes are looking at. If a series of gaze points is very close – in time and/or space – this gaze cluster constitutes a fixation, denoting a period where the eyes are locked towards an object. In our experiment, the subject was asked to concentrate on the image in front and therefore we can conclude that in between two saccades there is a fix. After detection of saccades, the time interval between two saccades are marked as fix, as shown in Figure 7.5.

7.3 SUMMARY

In this experiment, saccades and fixes were successfully segregated after applying appropriate noise removal and baseline drift removal techniques (Figure 7.5). Our future workproposal is to determine the direction of the eye

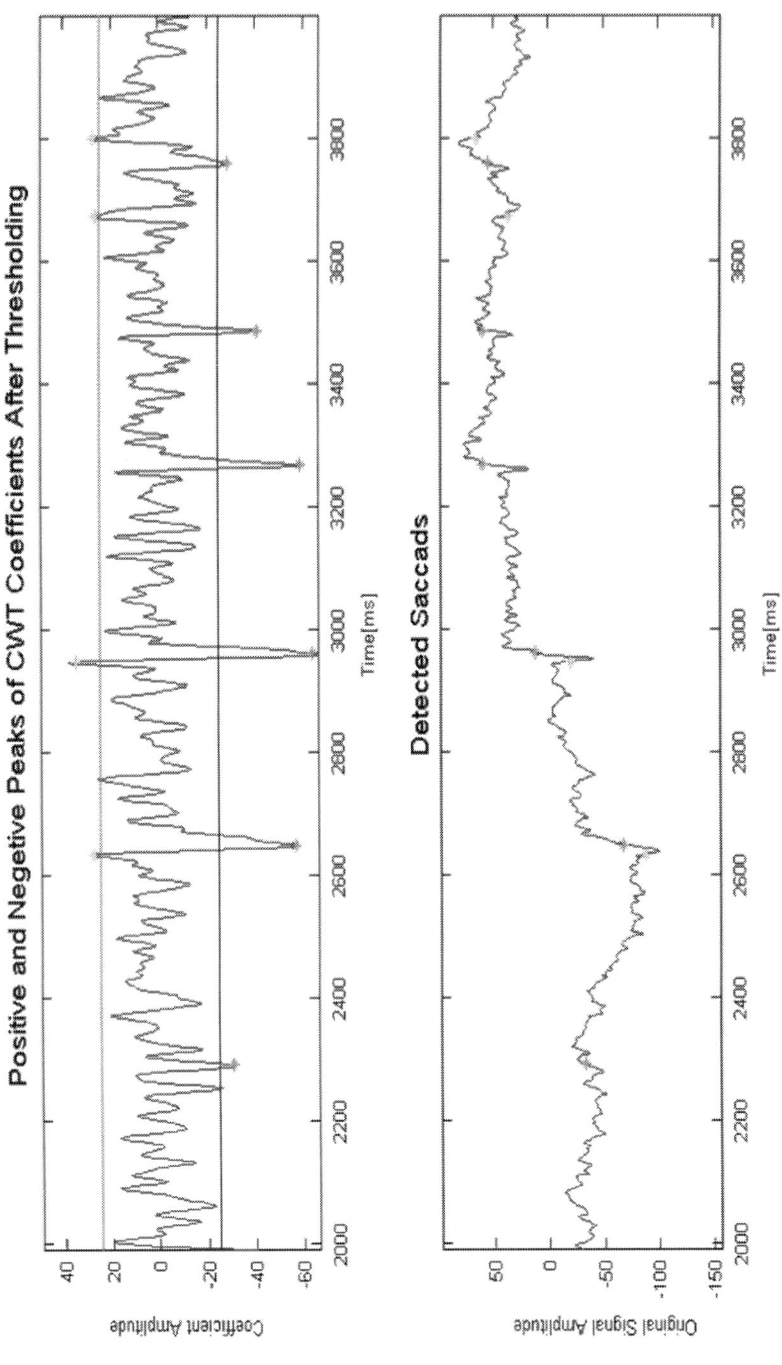

FIGURE 7.4 CWT coefficients of the signal with a threshold ±25 (top) and corresponding saccades (bottom).

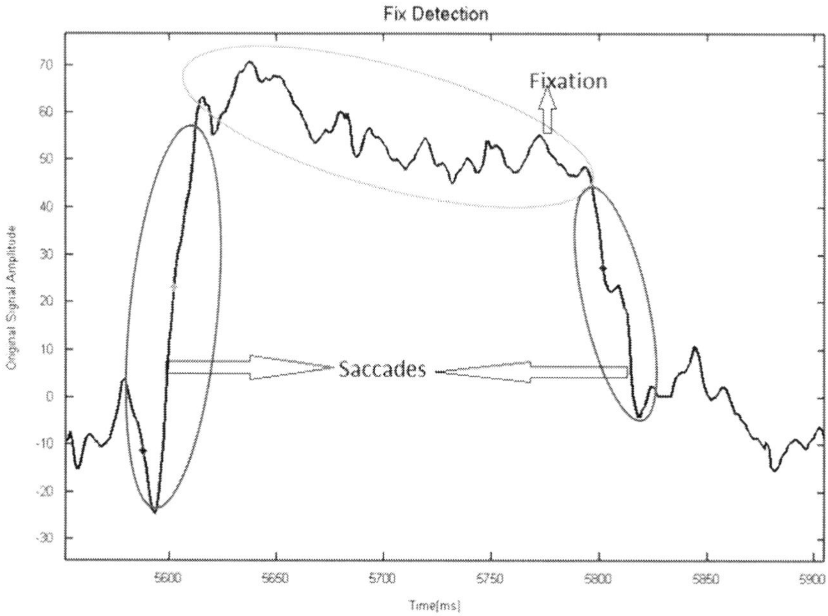

FIGURE 7.5 Demonstration of fix and saccades.

movement using detected saccades and plot a graph for further analysis. With the detected fixes, we also propose to detect the presence of P300 event-related potentials. This will relate to whether the subject is looking at an object of interest or not.

Exercises

1. What are saccade and fix artifacts in EOG signals? Give some physical significances of saccade and fixed in EOG data.
2. What are baseline drifting phenomena in EEG signals?
3. List different noise removal techniques for EEG signals.
4. Describe median filtering.
5. Describe wavelet denoising techniques in the context of EEG signals.
6. Describe the process of detection of saccade and fixation from EEG data.
7. Characterize fixation and how it manifests in time and space.

REFERENCES

Bulling, A, Ward, JA, Gellersen, H & Troster, G 2011 April, 'Eye movement analysis for activity recognition using electrooculography,' in *IEEE Transactions on Pattern Analysis and Machine Intelligence*, vol. 33, no. 4, pp. 741–753. doi:10.1109/TPAMI.2010.86

Du, P, Kibbe, WA & Lin, SM 2006 September 1, 'Improved peak detection in mass spectrum by incorporating continuous wavelet transform-based pattern matching,' *Bioinformatics*, vol. 22, no. 17, pp. 2059–2065. doi:10.1093/bioinformatics/btl355

Gao, J, Sultan, H, Hu, J & Tung, W 2010 March, 'Denoising nonlinear time series by adaptive filtering and wavelet shrinkage: A comparison,' in *IEEE Signal Processing Letters*, vol. 17, no. 3, pp. 237–240. doi:10.1109/LSP.2009.2037773.

Gupta, S & Singh, H 1996, 'Preprocessing EEG signals for direct human-system interface,' in *Proceedings IEEE International Joint Symposia on Intelligence and Systems*, Rockville, MD, USA, pp. 32–37. doi:10.1109/IJSIS.1996.565048

Henderson, JM & Andrew, H 2003, 'Eye movements and visual memory: Detecting changes to saccade targets in scenes,' *Perception & Psychophysics*, vol. 65, p. 58. doi:10.3758/BF03194783

Henn, V & Cohen, B 1973, 'Quantitative analysis of activity in eye muscle moto neurons during saccadic eye movements and positions of fixation,' *Journal of Neurophysiology*, vol. 36, no. 1, pp. 115–126, doi:10.1152/jn.1973.36.1.115

Nenadic, Z & Burdick, JW 2005 January, 'Spike detection using the continuous wavelet transform,' in *IEEE Transactions on Biomedical Engineering*, vol. 52, no. 1, pp. 74–87. doi:10.1109/TBME.2004.839800

Panigrahi, N, Roy, S, & Dey, A 2019a 'Saccade and fix detection from EoG signal,' IEEE iSES 2019, 16-18 Dec, 2019, NIT Rourkela, India.

Panigrahi, N, Roy, S, & Dey, A 2019b 'A method to detect blink from the EEG signal', *Intelligent Computing and Communication*. Singapore, Springer Nature. Chapter-1.1997/978-981-15-1084-7_24.

Patil, PB & Chavan, MS 2012, 'A wavelet based method for denoising of biomedical signal,' in *International Conference on Pattern Recognition, Informatics and Medical Engineering (PRIME-2012)*, Salem, Tamilnadu, pp. 278–283. doi:10.1109/ICPRIME.2012.6208358

8 Detection of P300 and Its Applications

8.1 INTRODUCTION

The human brain is the most complex organ of the body and it is at the center of the driving block of the human nervous system. In fact, more than 100 billion nerve cells are interconnected to build the functionality of the human brain. Such a complicated architecture allows the brain to control the body as well as carry out the executive functions, such as reasoning, processing thoughts, and planning for next tasks. Interestingly, electrophysiology and hemodynamic response are the two techniques that have been used to study this complex organ to understand the mechanism the brain applies to finish work. Typically, electrophysiological measurements are performed by placing electrodes or sensors on the biological tissue (Donchin et al 2000). In neuroscience and neuroengineering, the electrophysiological techniques are used for studying electrical properties by measuring the electrical activities of neurons in the form of an electroencephalogram (EEG). An EEG may be measured by two different approaches: invasive and non-invasive. Invasive procedures need a surgery to place the EEG sensor deep under the scalp. In comparison, non-invasive procedures place the electrodes on the scalp. One of the ways to study the brain is to stimulate it by presenting a paradigm.

The event-related potential (ERP) was first reported by Sutton (Klobassa et al 2009). An ERP is an electro-physiological response or electro-cortical potentials triggered by a stimulation and firing of neurons. A specific psychological event or a sensor can be employed to generate the stimulation. In general, visual, auditory, and tactile are three major sources of ERP stimulation. For instance, an ERP can be elicited by a surprise appearance of a character on a visual screen, or a "novel" tone presented over earphones, or by suddenly pressing a button by the subject, including myriad other events. The presented stimulus generates a detectable but time-delayed electrical wave in an EEG. An EEG is recorded starting from the time of presenting the stimulus to the time when the EEG settles down. Depending on the necessity, a simple detection method such as ensemble averaging or advanced processes such as linear discriminate analysis or support vector machine algorithms are applied on an EEG to measure the ERP. This chapter discusses the application of an ERP in the brain computer interface (BCI), where a P300 wave from the EEG is of particular interest. An ERP is time-locked to an event and appears as a series of positive and negative voltage fluctuation in the EEG, which are referred to as P300 components.

DOI: 10.1201/9781003241386-8

The secondary purpose of this chapter is to discuss various utilities and applications of P300 event-related potentials (ERPs). Also, we discuss how P300 has emerged as the artifact for a brain computer interface (BCI). Researchers and students will find this chapter interesting, with a preliminary description of a P300 ERP.

8.2 WHAT IS A P300 ARTIFACT IN AN EEG?

Sutton et al. in 1965 discovered the P300 signal. Since then, researchers in the field of ERP have analyzed it thoroughly. A P300 signal is an endogenous ERP. For most adults, in between the ages of 20 and 70, the latency range is 250–400 ms for auditory stimuli. The latency is defined as the speed of stimulus classification that results from discrimination of one event from another. Shorter latencies indicate superior mental performance compared to longer latencies. A P3 amplitude reflects stimulus information. It indicates that greater attention produces larger P3 waves.

The P300 is an event-related potential (ERP) endogenous component that has a positive deflection that occurs in the electroencephalogram (EEG) recorded from the scalp and typically elicited approximately 300 ms after the presentation of an infrequent stimulus (such as a visual, auditory, or somatosensory event) (Donchin et al 2000). The specific set of circumstances for eliciting a P300 is known as the oddball paradigm, which consists of presenting a target stimulus amid more frequent standard background stimuli. Under this paradigm, a P300, among other ERPs, is unconsciously elicited every time a subject's brain detects the target stimulus (the rare event). In fact, the P300 is a reasonable input signal, with desirable properties and stability to control brain computer interfaces (BCIs) (Klobassa et al 2009), applications requiring precise real-time detection as well as memory and computation optimization (Hoffmann et al 2008; Pires et al 2011). The feature vector dimensionality reduction has been a popular choice to achieve these goals within the BCI community because it decreases the complexity of classifiers (Krusienski et al 2008). A reduced P300 amplitude is an indication of the broad neurobiological vulnerability that determines disorders within the externalizing spectrum.

The features of a P300 have been represented in time, frequency, time-frequency, and shape domains by using, among others, wavelet transform (Bostanov 2004), genetic algorithms (Atum et al 2010), and common spatial patterns (Krusienski et al 2007). Additionally, the approaches more commonly used for P300 classification are linear discriminate analysis (LDA), step-wise linear discriminate analysis (Krusienski et al 2006), and support vector machines (Kaper et al 2004).

8.3 CHARACTERISTICS OF P300 WAVEFORMS

A P300 is a form of visually evoked potential (VEP) and a P300 ERP (Figure 8.1) is embedded within the EEG signal recordable from the scalp of the

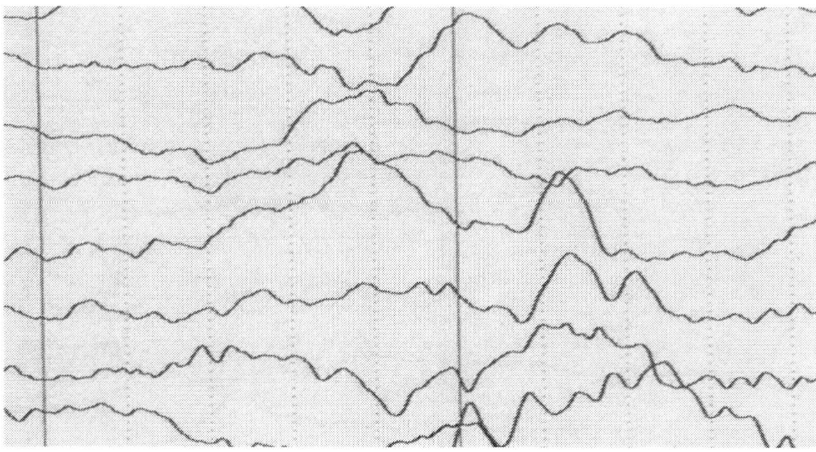

FIGURE 8.1 P300 signal with high peaks in the EEG.

human brain. The P300 positive deflection occurs in the EEG about 300 ms after an eliciting stimulus is delivered, which is the major reason it is termed a P300. Depending on the components' appearance following the eliciting event, the P300 can be divided into two parts: exogenous and endogenous. Out of the 300 ms duration of the waveform, early (exogenous) components are distributed over the first 150 ms. The longer latency (endogenous) components elicit after 150 ms. The latency of the P300 wave can be within the range from 250 to 750 ms. Research has established that a P300 is elicited by the decision making or learning that a rare event has registered by the brain. Some things appear to be learned by the brain if and only if they are surprising. The variable latency is associated with the difficulty of the decision making. In addition, the largest P300 responses are obtained over the parietal zone of the human head while it is attenuated with the electrodes that are gradually placed farther from this area.

8.4 HOW TO GENERATE OR INDUCE A P300

To generate the P300 ERP, three different types of paradigms are used: (1) single-stimulus, (2) oddball, and (3) three-stimulus paradigms. In each case, the subject is instructed to follow the occurrence of the target by pressing a button or mentally counting. Figure 8.2 presents these paradigms. The single-stimulus paradigm irregularly presents just one type of stimuli or target with zero occurrence of any other type of target. A typical oddball paradigm can be presented to the subject with a computer screen, a group of light-emitting diodes (LEDs), or other medium to generate a sequence of events that can be categorized into two classes: frequently presented standard (non target or irrelevant) and rarely presented target stimuli. In an oddball paradigm, two events are presented with different probabilities in a random order, but only the irregular

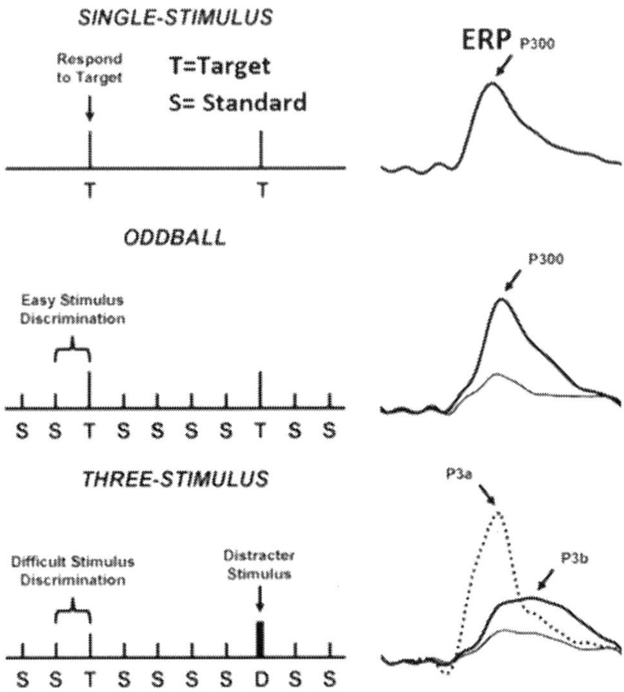

FIGURE 8.2 Schematic account of three paradigms: single-stimulus (top), oddball (middle), and three-stimulus (bottom). Elicited ERP is presented at the right.

and rare event (the oddball event) embosses the P300 peak into the EEG about 300 ms after the stimulus onset. The three-stimulus paradigm is a modified oddball task that includes a non-target distracter (infrequent non-target) stimuli in addition to target and standard stimuli. The distractor elicits a P3a that is large over the frontal/central area. In contrast, a target elicits a P3b (P300), which is maximum over the parietal electrode sites. Though P3a and P3b are sub-components of P300, P3a is dominant in the frontal/central lobe with a shorter latency.

8.5 P300 DETECTION

Detection of a P300 requires the subject to properly recognize the stimulus event to generate a strong and perceivable P300 ERP. A noticeable P300 amplitude is also critical for information transfer, which might not be possible if the stimulation is presented too fast or the targets appear too frequently (Kaper et al 2004). It is important to design a BCI paradigm with easily discriminable stimuli. A BCI should be adjustable to the users' adaptability of signal detection by controlling the stimulus presentation at a slower rate, brighter intensity, or with otherwise increasing perceptibility. Studies also show that target-to-target interval (TTI) plays an important role in evoking a larger P300 ERP. If the overall BCI paradigm presents the stimulation at a constant rate, targets with low probability result in longer TTI, which is also a useful means to obtain perceivable P300 amplitude. In sum, for a stronger P300 ERP, the BCI system should maintain a minimum probability or maximum TTI. Unfortunately, such an action reduces the frequency of the target stimulation and, thereby, reduces the overall system speed. This trade-off has been explored in several early BCI studies. It is evident that due to the nature of P300 ERP generation, a P300 amplitude can be increased by incorporating high temporal uncertainty. In this case, subjects are completely unaware of the exact time when the stimulation occurs. A few articles reported that a P300 amplitude becomes larger for familiar or learned items. For example, if a list of characters is presented to a subject repeatedly, P300 amplitudes for repeated characters (which are recalled by the subject) are higher than the characters that are forgotten by the user.

In addition, there are several other factors which should be considered for P300 detection. Among these are attentional blink, which occurs in case the intervals between two different targets become less than 500 ms; repetition blindness, which leaves the second target unnoticed if two identical targets flash at intervals between 100 and 500 ms; and habituation, which makes a faint P300 amplitude due to the repeated presentation of the same stimulus. Apart from this, human factors such as motivation, fatigue, and user comfort ability affect the performance and accuracy of the P300 BCI, which should be considered in the design of paradigms.

8.6 SIGNAL PROCESSING METHODS

A P300-based BCI measures EEG signals from the human scalp and processes them in real time to detect a P300 ERP that reflects the subject's intent. As noted earlier, P300-evoked potential is elicited as positive EEG peaks in reaction to infrequent or irregular appearance of stimuli. As the EEG signals are typically in the order of 100 μV, an appropriate signal processing strategy is critical in revealing the electrical information and relevant complex issues in relation to the distinctive cognitive functions. Moreover, optimization of accuracy in a P300 detection and enhancement of the system speed heavily depends on a suitable signal processing scheme.

An EEG-based BCI system can have three stages to process signals: pre-processing, feature extraction, and detection and classification of a P300. Pre-processing is accomplished after data acquisition but before extracting any feature. Pre-processing is an important step that leaves the significant information intact while amplifying EEG signals and simplifying subsequent processing operations. It is also important to note that the classifier performance depends greatly on an efficient data pre-processing stage. Signal strengthening ensures signal quality by improving the so-called signal-to-noise ratio (SNR). The presence of background noise may bury the interesting brain patterns into the rest of the signal, making it difficult to detect a P300 response, resulting in a bad or small SNR. On the other hand, a P300 detection and classification becomes easier when the input EEG signal has a high SNR. After acquiring the EEG signal from microelectrodes or macroelectrodes, the electrical information is amplified by a factor as high as 5,000–10,000 and converted from an analog to a digital signal. Though analog to digital A/D conversion can be done at a rate of a few GHz, the human brain does not operate that fast to justify such a high sampling frequency. EEG data is typically sampled at 256 Hz, which satisfies the Nyquist sampling theorem as this rate is larger than two times the maximum frequency generated by cognitive actions, yet low enough to avoid irrelevant data. To realize the high SNR, band-pass filtering is utilized to remove the DC bias and high-frequency noise. Sometimes researchers also combine transformation and filtering techniques and apply them to remove or abate signal components that are not of interest for the application. As AC current is usually of 50–60 Hz, depending on the particular living zone of the globe, a notch filter at either 50–60 Hz is used to remove the powerline effect on an EEG. During the filter setup, it should be kept in mind that certain types of artifacts occur at known frequencies and cognitive activity usually limits itself in the 3–40 Hz range.

Once the EEG is preprocessed, a variety of approaches can be applied to extract the features and classify the P300 ERP. A calibration session is exploited to develop these feature vectors. Before the classification test and actual use of the P300 BCI, the classifier is trained and supervised using a classification algorithm and the feature vectors are labeled as "target" and "non-target." On the other hand, during the classification task, the feature vectors corresponding to known stimuli are submitted to a trained classifier. The trained classifier discriminates the brain response best resembling a target stimulus from a non-target stimulus. In the case of a P300 Speller, the classifier detects the letter with a maximum probability.

Different methods have been employed for feature extraction, such as discrete wavelet transform, independent component analysis, and principal component analysis. As stated earlier, extracted features are given as input to the EEG classifiers for P300 ERP identification and classification applying different classification methods. Linear discriminate analysis (LDA) is a popular pattern classification technique used by Guger et al. Step-wise linear discriminate analysis (SWDA) has evolved from the LDA classification method that uses only selective features. Farwell and Donchin used SWDA to classify the ERP using individual averages for rows and columns of a 6 × 6 row/column paradigm. Some classification methods apply machine learning techniques for the P300 detection, such as support vector machines (SVMs). A SVM takes advantage of small data size to give high throughput at a high transfer rate. However, LDA outperforms SVM classifiers for the P300 detection if the input data is comparatively larger in size. Moreover, many BCI groups have exercised their study with other classifiers such as Bayesian linear discriminate analysis (BLDA), Pearson's correlation method (PCM), linear support vector machine (LSVM), and Gaussian support vector machine (GSVM). Although different features and

TABLE 8.1
Summary of the signal processing methods used to detect a P300 from an EEG signal

Methods	System Performance
Discrete wavelet transform (DWT)	Accuracy >90%, 6 × 6 targets on the menu; 36 feature vectors; feature vectors were continually ranked and either a correlation/threshold was used to select a cell
Genetic algorithm (GA)	Variable accuracy, 34%~90% high resource consumption; possible premature convergence
Bayesian analysis, Bayesian linear discriminant analysis (BLDA)	Feature vector is labeled to the class to which it has the highest probability with 95% false positive classification accuracy
Linear discriminant analysis (LDA); simple, low computation	Accuracy for the able-bodied subjects was on average close to 100% and the best classification accuracy for disabled subjects
Support vector machine (SVM); linear and nonlinear (Gaussian) modalities, faster processing	96.5% accuracy
Maximum likelihood (ML)	Feature detection using a priori knowledge; accuracy 90% with a communication rate of 4.19 symbols/min

classifiers have been compared, there has not been a comprehensive comparison of all different feature extractions and classification methods applied to the same data set. The most frequently used signal processing methods have been described in Table 8.1 with reference to the relevant study.

8.7 APPLICATIONS OF P300 SYSTEMS

A P300 BCI is particularly suitable for select applications. For instance, the most typical application of a P300 BCI is a P300 speller. In such an arrangement, the visual paradigm is made up of a matrix consisting of letters of the alphabet. Depending on the requirement, a speller can be optimized for quick selection or accuracy of the spelled letters. Similarly, other P300 BCI investigations have made extensive progress to develop other attractive applications such as painting artwork, controlling a smart home, designing games, stroke rehabilitation, lie detection, and furnishing Internet tasks. However, recognizing the importance of a P300 speller, a detailed description of a P300 speller is presented in the following sections. An overview of some popular applications of a P300 is depicted in Figure 8.3.

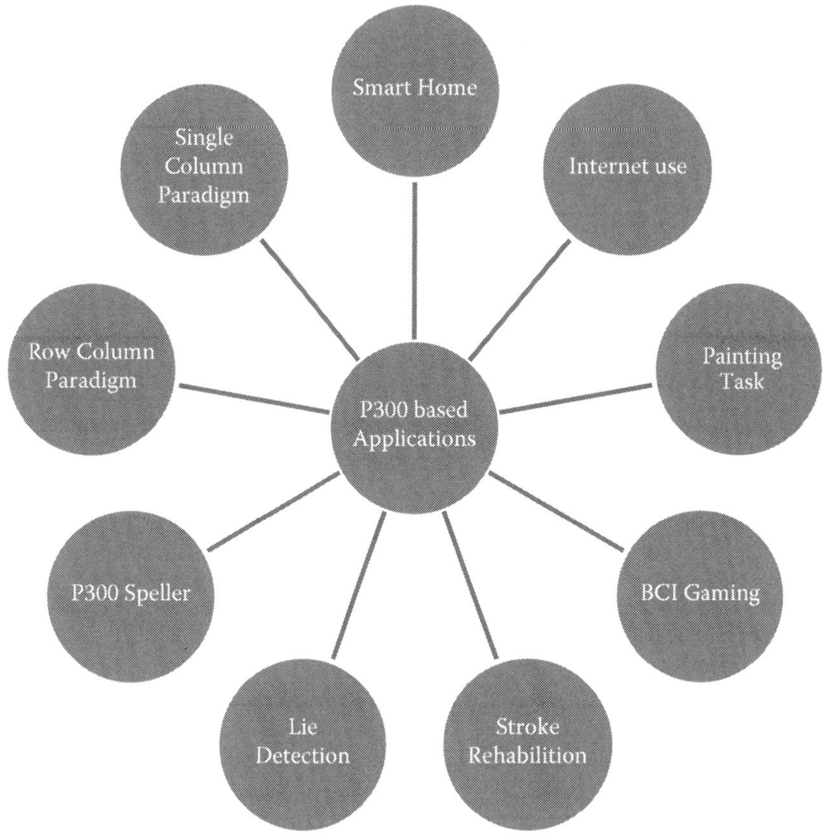

FIGURE 8.3 Popular applications of a P300.

8.7.1 Smart Home

A smart home populates different electronic devices that can be controlled using a P300 BCI. A virtual reality–based smart home was the test-bed of such a BCI application. This BCI system was allowed to execute a group of modest controlling commands such as moving the cart or wheelchair, receiving or making phone calls, operating a television, switching the light on and off, playing a song in a multimedia player, or controlling doors and windows.

8.7.2 Internet Use

A P300 BCI can be used to select the Internet keys to provide assistance to amyotrophic lateral sclerosis (ALS) patients browsing websites. Subjects can surf through Internet pages and select the desired links to browse the Internet or read the news using the P300 activation.

8.7.3 Painting Tasks

It was observed by researchers that performing natural tasks brings a better quality to life in ALS patients. A P300 BCI application known as "brain painting" (BP) offers a medium of entertainment for patients by improving their playful mood.

8.7.4 BCI Gaming

A P300 BCI has been used to design a paradigm to control simple games that do not require strong time constraints, such as playing chess. Other popular games using a P300 BCI are MindGame, Bacteria Hunt, Brain Invaders, etc. In MindGame, the user's move depends on the brain response; if a P300 ERP is stronger, the game character can move a larger distance. In Bacteria Hunt, users can change the color of the image, or enlarge or rotate it. Similarly, in Brain Invaders, the user needs to select an appropriate target arm to destroy the aliens, which makes the game interesting to the video game players. As no training is required to start playing simple P300 BCI games as mentioned here, it can be useful to familiarize individuals to the BCI tools. In fact, proper design to utilize the P300 wave's strong dependence on attention would allow the scientists to study attention training and effects of engaging in a particular task.

8.7.5 Stroke Rehabilitation

One of the sufferings of post-stroke patients is that they would like to say what they want but the trouble of cortical circuits will not allow them to express it through natural motor pathways. A P300 BCI paradigm was used to provide a communication channel to the participants diagnosed with post-stroke aphasia. A P300 BCI not only allowed them to activate their language circuits, but also made their post-stroke recovery faster.

8.7.6 Lie Detection

Different brain regions work together and generate activities to process deceptive information that elicits a P300 ERP in the brain signal. The concealed information can be identified through the concealed information test (CIT). Most of the earlier experiments with lie detectors used just a few channels, limiting the number of EEG features to classify these two types of information. These studies mostly used an oddball paradigm using three different types of stimuli: target, probe, and irrelevant. Like a typical P300-based system, the targets are presented rarel,y though they are usually made of irrelevant items that are presented in the paradigm to ensure participants' cooperation in discriminating the target items from others. On the contrary, the irrelevant items are presented frequently, but they are neither related to the criminal act nor related to the experimental task. The underlying principle of the item is that subjects will have different responses to stimuli according to their crime-relevant status. The probes are the critical detail stimuli under investigation that appear infrequently. Probes elicit a P300 only for subjects who are knowledgeable or are deceiving the information. Otherwise, they act similarly as irrelevant for the subject. However, to ensure reliable differences between liars and truth-tellers, it is important to engage multiple channels, resulting in ERP features from different brain areas. One study investigated the functional connectivity of the brain network under a deception condition. They found the correlation between different EEG signals from multiple channels to understand the interactions between the brain regions and functional connectivity. Their results suggest that incorporation of additional features helps separate the innocent group from the liars with about 90% accuracy.

8.7.7 P300 Speller

Perhaps the most important and popular use of a P300 BCI is a P300 speller. A BCI speller has been utilized as a communication tool for the last two decades by people suffering from various neuromuscular disorders such as ALS, brainstem stroke, brain or spinal cord injury, cerebral palsy, muscular dystrophy, multiple sclerosis, and other impaired patients who are unable to use the normal neuronal pathways. Persistent research in a BCI to improve the accuracy and speed of a P300 speller has resulted in numerous P300 stimuli presentation paradigms. They are discussed in detail in the following sections.

8.7.7.1 Row/Column (RC) Paradigm

The Farwell and Donchin matrix speller paradigm was the first BCI row-column speller (Figure 8.4). They used an alphabetical square matrix interface to produce a P300 in an EEG. Rows and columns of this 6 × 6 matrix were constructed with alphanumeric characters. These characters are flashed randomly following either a row or a column and the subject is asked to mentally count the number of times that the attended character is flashed. During the brain signal measurement in the parietal area, the P300 ERP appears in an EEG as an evoked response. However, the non-flashing rows and columns do not generate a P300. Due to the nature of the stimulation mechanism and to increase the accuracy of detection, the P300 system requires multiple trials to reach an acceptable accuracy. In practice, the non-target rows also generate a P300 for a very short amount of time but the amplitude is too faint to detect. The computational device can determine the target row and column after averaging several P300 ERP responses. Due to the averaging task, it may take a longer time to detect a character. In general, reducing the number of characters would eliminate the longer detection time but not without a loss in spelling character options. So far, this is the most used and discussed P300 speller in the BCI community.

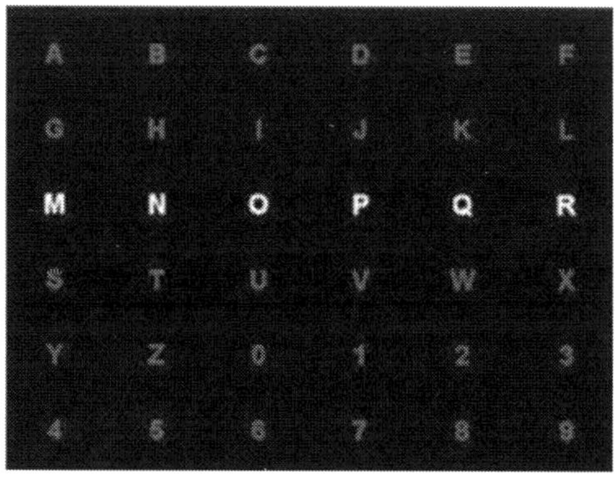

FIGURE 8.4 The row-column (RC) paradigm. One row (MNOPQR) is flashing.

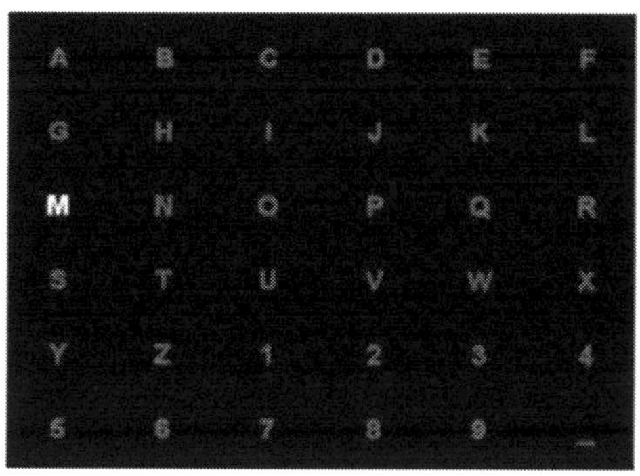

FIGURE 8.5 Single character (SC) paradigm: single character (M) is flashed.

8.7.7.2 Single Character (SC) Paradigm

This is possibly one of the simplest spellers designed so far. It randomly flashes one character at a time with very short interflash interval (Figure 8.5). This paradigm also uses a 6 × 6 alphanumeric matrix like the RC paradigm. It was reported that the RC paradigm takes less time than the SC paradigm to flash all the characters at least once. Nevertheless, it was noticed that if the number of flashes is constant, the SC speller produces a stronger P300 ERP than the RC speller.

8.8 SUMMARY

An ERP is a change in voltage that is time-locked to a specific sensory, motor, or cognitive event. An ERP provides a distinctive pattern as an indication of how the stimulus is processed. Many BCI applications have been developed based on an ERP as a response to a stimulus. Among these, a P300-based BCI is the most prominent ERP BCI. Over the last two decades, countless P300 BCI works have exploded beyond laboratory experiments with the help of modern high-speed computational and sensor technologies.

P300 applications range from the potential improvement of lifestyle to financial benefits. In fact, fundamental research on recording hardware, signal processing methods, stimulus presentation parameters, supporting interaction paradigm, and neurophysiology will further refine the P300-based BCI design. Though a BCI design is accomplished by keeping a specific application in mind, further insightful study and research can revive opportunities toward exploring other usable areas that are still not unearthed. This chapter has covered several aspects and applications of P300 ERPs in BCI research. The interfacing paradigm of a P300 BCI can be designed to capture the ERP-evoked potentials in a manner so that many human factors are properly taken care of to diminish their overall negative impact. Many new applications are also emerging with an efficient design of the control interface and associated signal processing scheme.

Exercises

1. What are P300 artifacts in an EEG? What are the characteristics of a P300 signal?
2. What are the applications of a P300 signal?
3. What is an ERP (event-related potential) and how is an ERP manifested in an EEG?
4. How do you induce a P300 or generate a P300 in a subject?
5. What is a different feature extraction method used to extract features from a P300 signal?
6. What is a P300 speller and what is it used for?
7. What is a row-column paradigm?

REFERENCES

Atum, Y, Gareis, I, Gentiletti, G, Acevedo, R & Rufiner, L 2010 September, 'Genetic feature selection to optimally detect P300 in brain computer interfaces,' in *Proceedings of the IEEE Engineering in Medicine and Biology 27th Annual Conference (EMBC'10)*, Buenos Aires, Argentina, pp. 3289–3292.

Bostanov, V 2004, 'BCI competition 2003-data sets Ib and IIb: feature extraction from event-related brain potentials with the continuous wavelet transform and the t-value scalogram,' *IEEE Transactions on Biomedical Engineering*, vol. 51, no. 6, pp. 1057–1061. doi:10.1109/tbme.2004.826702

Donchin, E, Spencer, KM & Wijesinghe, R 2000, 'The mental prosthesis: Assessing the speed of a P300-based brain-computer interface,' *IEEE Transactions on Rehabilitation Engineering*, vol. 8, no. 2, pp. 174–179. doi:10.1109/86.847808

Hoffmann, U, Vesin, J-M, Ebrahimi, T & Diserens, K 2008, 'An efficient P300-based brain-computer interface for disabled subjects,' *Journal of Neuroscience Methods*, vol. 167, no. 1, pp. 115–125. doi:10.1016/j.jneumeth.2007.03.005

Kaper, M, Meinicke, P, Grossekathoefer, U, Lingner, T & Ritter, H 2004, 'BCI competition 2003-data set IIb: Support vector machines for the P300 speller paradigm,'

IEEE Transactions on Biomedical Engineering, vol. 51, no. 6, pp. 1073–1076. doi:10.1109/tbme.2004.826698

Klobassa, DS, Vaughan, TM, Brunner, P, et al. 2009, 'Toward a high-throughput auditory P300-based brain-computer interface,' *Clinical Neurophysiology*, vol. 120, no. 7, pp. 1252–1261. doi:10.1016/j.clinph.2009.04.019

Krusienski, DJ, Sellers, EW, Cabestaing, F, et al. 2006, 'A comparison of classification techniques for the P300 Speller', *Journal of Neural Engineering*, vol. 3, no. 4, pp. 299–305. doi:10.1088/1741-2560/3/4/007.

Krusienski, DJ, Sellers, EW, McFarland, DJ, Vaughan, TM & Wolpaw, JR 2008, 'Toward enhanced P300 speller performance,' *Journal of Neuroscience Methods*, vol. 167, no. 1, pp. 15–21. doi:10.1016/j.jneumeth.2007.07.017

Krusienski, DJ, Sellers, EW & Vaughan, TM 2007 May, 'Common spatio-temporal patterns for the P300 speller,' in *Proceedings of the 3rd International IEEE EMBS Conference on Neural Engineering (CNE '07)*, Kohala Coast, Hawaii, USA, pp. 421–424.

Pires, G, Nunes, U & Castelo-Branco, M 2011, 'Statistical spatial filtering for a P300-based BCI: Tests in able-bodied, and patients with cerebral palsy and amyotrophic lateral sclerosis,' *Journal of Neuroscience Methods*, vol. 195, no. 2, pp. 270–281. doi:10.1016/j.jneumeth.2010.11.016

9 Brain Computer Interface Using P300

Advances in cognitive neuroscience and brain imaging technologies have enabled the brain to directly interface with the computer. This technique is called a brain computer interface (BCI). This ability is made possible through the use of sensors that can monitor some of the physical processes that occur inside the brain. Researchers have used these kinds of technologies to build brain computer interfaces (BCIs). Computers or communication devices can be controlled by using the signals produced in the brain. This is very useful for all those who are not able to communicate with the outside world directly. They can easily forecast their emotions or feelings using this technology. In a BCI, we use oddball paradigms to generate event-related potentials (ERPs), like the P300 wave, on targets that have been selected by the user.

The basic principle of a BCI is to detect the presence of a P300 in the electroencephalogram (EEG). Then, to classify the combination of different P300 signals for determining the right kind of task. In this chapter, both parts i.e., the classification as well as characterization part, are presented in a simple and lucid way. The raw data was processed through MATLAB® software and the corresponding feature matrices were obtained. Several techniques such as normalization, feature extraction, and feature reduction were carried out.

9.1 INTRODUCTION

Brain computer interfaces (BCIs) are tools for controlling computers and other devices without using muscular activity, but employing user-controlled variations in signals recorded from the user's brain. One of the most efficient noninvasive BCIs is based on the P300 wave of the brain's response to stimuli and is therefore referred to as the P300 BCI. Many modifications of this BCI have been proposed to further improve the BCI's characteristics or to better adapt the BCI to various applications. However, in the original P300 BCI and in all of its modifications, the spatial positions of stimuli were fixed relative to each other, which can impose constraints on designing applications controlled by this BCI. We designed and tested a P300 BCI with stimuli presented on objects that were freely and randomly presented on a screen. The process of a P300 BCI is depicted in Figure 9.1.

DOI: 10.1201/9781003241386-9

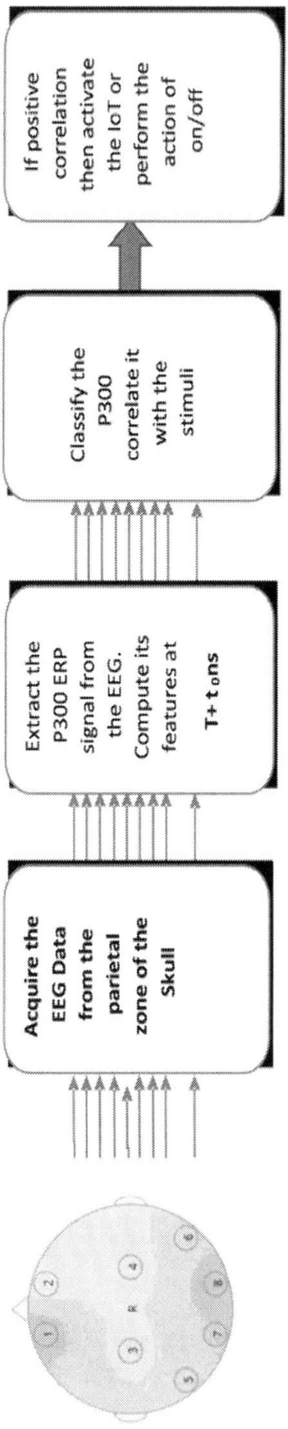

FIGURE 9.1 The plot of a P300-based brain computer interface with stimuli on moving objects.

9.2 THE P300 BCI AND MOVEMENT

A brain computer interface (BCI) is a communication system that provides the user with the ability to send messages or commands to the external world without using the brain's normal output pathways, i.e., without using peripheral nerves and muscles (Wolpaw et al 2002). BCIs are primarily developed as an assistive technology to help people with severe paralysis, but this technology is also increasingly used by healthy people, especially in video games (Plass-Oude Bos et al 2010). Within BCI technology, fundamentally new aspects of interaction between the brain and computers emerge because this technology provides completely new "output pathways" for the brain (Wolpaw 2007). The operation of these pathways typically requires conscious control, but interestingly, unconscious BCI control is also possible (Kaplan et al 2005).

Currently, the most commonly used BCI is likely the P300-based BCI (the P300 BCI) (Mak et al 2011). In this BCI, available commands are coded by stimuli presented at different locations and times. The user attends the stimuli presented at a location associated with a desired command and ignores the stimuli presented at all other locations, which are associated with different commands. The BCI analyzes the user's electroencephalogram (EEG), which is typically recorded non-invasively (from the scalp), and can recognize which stimuli are attended because this behavior results in a specific pattern in his or her EEG. As soon as the BCI recognizes one of the stimuli as attended, the system executes the command that corresponds to this stimulus (Figure 9.2).

All existing variations of the visual P300 BCI design share a common feature: the positions at which stimuli are presented are spatially fixed. The original version of the P300 BCI (Farwell & Donchin 1988) was developed for spelling, and for this purpose, it was convenient to organize the stimulus positions in a matrix (see Figure 9.3(b)). Most of the current P300 BCIs are also spellers, and it is surprising that the matrix design still prevails. Additionally, various new applications of the P300 BCI in which the matrix is used as a "control panel" for entering commands, e.g., for robots or wheelchairs, are common. However, the matrix design is not always appropriate because more freedom is often needed in positioning the locations to be attended for entering commands. Moreover, at least in several applications, *moving stimulus positions* may be useful.

Consider, for example, a user of an assistive or telepresence mobile robot controlled with a P300 BCI. To enter a command, the user must concentrate for a considerable time on stimuli presented on a control panel. After recognition of the command by the BCI, the user's attention must switch to a remotely located robot to check how the command is executed. The attention then must return to the control panel to enter the next command. These multiple attention shifts not only pose an unnecessary burden on the attention system (already heavily loaded with the task of attending the stimuli) but also make more dynamic control difficult, e.g., in such situations that require fast canceling of the current operation if an error occurs. Placing the control panel on robotic devices or even

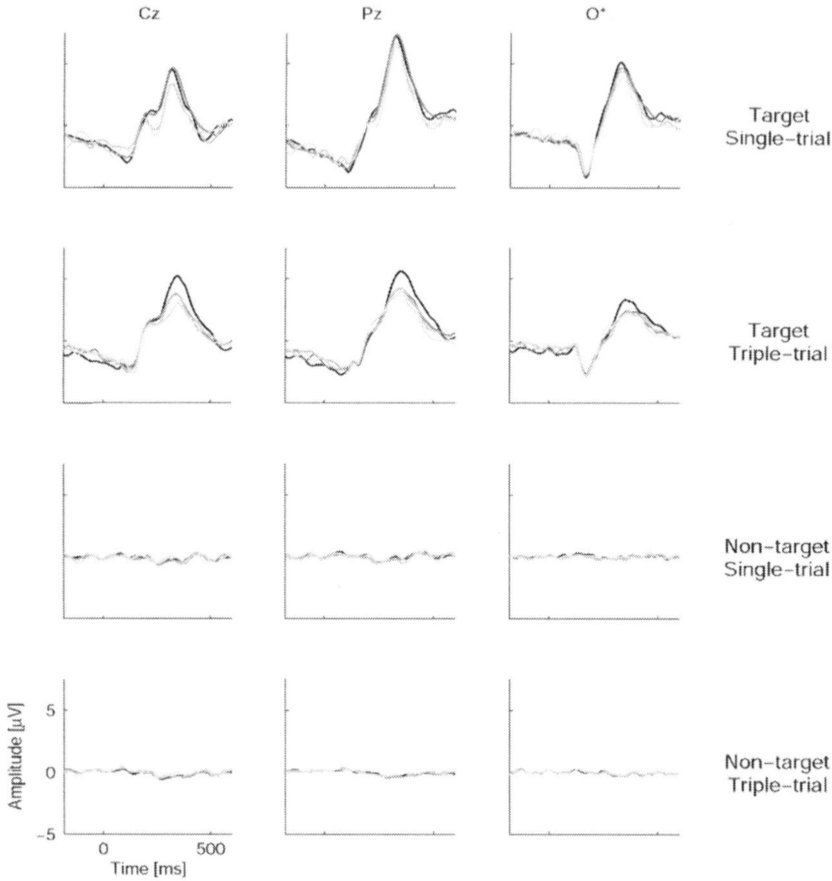

FIGURE 9.2 Four-session single-trial and Triple-Trial tests with a Game-like task.

placing several of the panel's elements on separate moving parts of such devices might be a more efficient solution, at least in certain cases.

Video games are another prospective application to which the standard P300 BCI is not well suited due to this BCI's static design. At least several of the P300 BCI's characteristics are certainly suited to gaming applications: the BCI does not require prior training for the user to start operating it, and a very high percentage of people are able to use it (Guger et al 2009). Surprisingly, among the many BCI games already proposed (see, e.g., Plass-Oude Bos et al 2010 for a review), only few are based on the P300 BCI technology (Kaplan et al 2013). The shortcomings of the P300 BCI in its application in gaming are currently being successfully overcome by various means (Kaplan et al 2013). One of the possible answers to the question of why BCI game developers are reluctant to use the P300 BCI is its static design; games without movement on the screen are relatively rare and often not very engaging.

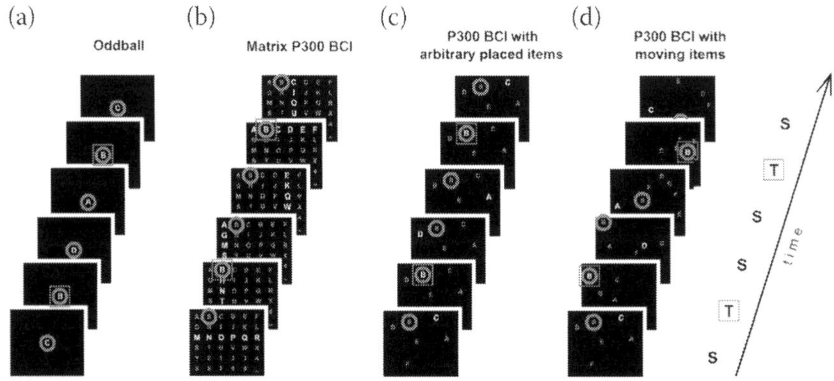

FIGURE 9.3 Spatial organization of stimulus in the P300 BCI compared with the oddball paradigm. (a) Visual oddball paradigm. (b) Matrix ("classical") P300 BCI layout with stimuli grouped into rows and columns. (c) P300 BCI layout with fixed arbitrary stimulus positions and single-cell presentation mode (without grouping). (d) P300 BCI layout with moving stimulus positions and single-cell presentation mode (a design used in this study). S, standards (non-target stimuli). T, targets (target stimuli). In these examples, a flashing letter *B* is the target stimulus. Note that the content at the location that should be attended (marked with a grey circle) significantly varies with sequential presentations in the oddball paradigm (a) (both targets and standards are presented there), whereas in the P300 BCI (b, c, d), the attended location can be in one of two states only (target stimulus on/off; the standards are presented at other locations).

Stimuli are essential to the P300 BCI. To avoid the division of spatial attention between an important game element and a stimulus, the element and the stimulus should have the same or at least overlapping spatial locations (Kaplan et al 2013). Further integration of the BCI into a game and further support for maintaining attention to the same location can be ensured if the result of the command entered through the BCI acts upon the elements (e.g., enlarges, transforms, multiplies, or destroys the elements) (Kaplan et al 2013).

A P300 BCI design that is vivid and flexible compared with standard matrix-based approaches appears to have already been achieved by BCI developers, who proposed presenting stimuli on freely placed virtual objects (e.g., Bayliss 2003; Donnerer & Steed 2010; Yuksel et al 2011) or even highlighting real objects as stimuli (Mak et al 2011; Yuksel et al 2010, 2011). However, even in these BCIs, the stimulus objects were static, as in all P300 BCI-controlled games described in the literature to date. This feature is a serious drawback of the P300 BCI games compared with games based on other BCIs, such as motor imagery BCI, in which the movement of an attended object is relatively common.

In most popular video games, the visual elements on which attention is focused are typically not static, but moving, and that movement plays an important role in making these games engaging. It is difficult to create an attractive game on the basis of the static control panel of the standard P300 BCI.

However, the P300 BCI can be used without prior training by a very high percentage of people (Guger et al 2009), unlike nearly all other BCIs. This feature appears to be particularly important in such a potentially highly marketable application as video games.

It therefore seems logical to combine the P300 BCI with the free movement of key visual elements in games by attaching the stimuli to these elements. However, such a step has not been made to date.

Movement of the P300 BCI stimulus matrix was studied in several cases: in our experiment, targeting the possible influence of movement on an event-related potential (ERP) and BCI accuracy (Shishkin et al 2011); in a P300 BCI game (Congedo et al 2011); and in BCI-controlled wheelchairs, in which the matrix position was not fixed relative to the environment in which the wheelchair moved (e.g., Rebsamen et al 2010). However, in all of these studies, the stimulus positions were fixed relative to each other, which seems to be a serious constraint for game designers and, in certain cases, for designers of BCI control for robotic assistive devices.

Modifications of the P300 BCI with moving stimuli have been proposed (Guan, Chen et al 2005; Guo, Hong et al 2008; Hong et al 2009; Liu et al 2010,. In all of these cases, the initiation of movement and/or the appearance of a moving stimulus were used as stimuli or as a part of a complex stimulus. However, all of these studies described paradigms in which each stimulus moved within a small area, and most importantly, the spatial positions at which the stimuli were presented did not change significantly from trial to trial. Thus, the basic static spatial design of the P300 BCI was unchanged.

To the best of our knowledge, no journal publications to date have explored the feasibility of a P300 BCI in which the stimuli are presented at positions that move significantly relative to each other.

In the following sections, we will introduce the P300 BCI in more detail and provide arguments showing that existing knowledge was not sufficient to predict whether the P300 BCI would work efficiently when the stimulus positions move relative to each other. Therefore, an experimental study was needed to test the P300 BCI under this condition. We then explain additional goals of our study, i.e., testing the possible effects of multisession practice with such a BCI under other conditions and in single-trial and triple-trial stimulation modes.

9.2.1 Functioning of the P300 BCI

The P300 BCI was designed by Farwell and Donchin (Farwell & Donchin 1988) to send commands from the brain to a computer using the P300 wave. This wave, which is also referred to as the P3 wave, is a large positive wave observed in human ERPs approximately 300 ms or longer after the beginning of a stimulus. The wave is elicited when the stimulus is unpredictable or not fully predictable and automatically attracts attention or is voluntarily attended because it requires a certain response, whether overt (motor) or covert (purely mental). In a BCI, such a response can only be covert and has the form of silent counting or just "mental noting" of the stimulus. Later, other ERP components were also shown to be useful in the framework of a BCI. The standard task used in psychophysiology to elicit the P300 is referred to as the "oddball paradigm." In this task, different events are sequentially presented to a participant. In the most standard design of the oddball paradigm, several of these events (the targets) are less frequent and require a motor or mental response, whereas the more frequent events (the standards) require no action and can be ignored.

The process of a BCI (brain computer interface) as a system to control IoT-based devices and generate decisions that will drive the device is given in the block diagram (Figure 9.4). The main steps describe how the P300 signal is elicited in the brain of the subject by presenting an external stimuli. The stimuli is based on a oddball experiment, which is a row-column syndrome. The EEG signal from the parietal zone of the scalp is collected, corresponding to the stimuli. The signal collected is passed through a notch filter to remove the signal error. Further, the signal is boosted to a higher power spectrum for convenience of processing. The α, β, ϒ, δ, and P300 EEG waves were segregated from the

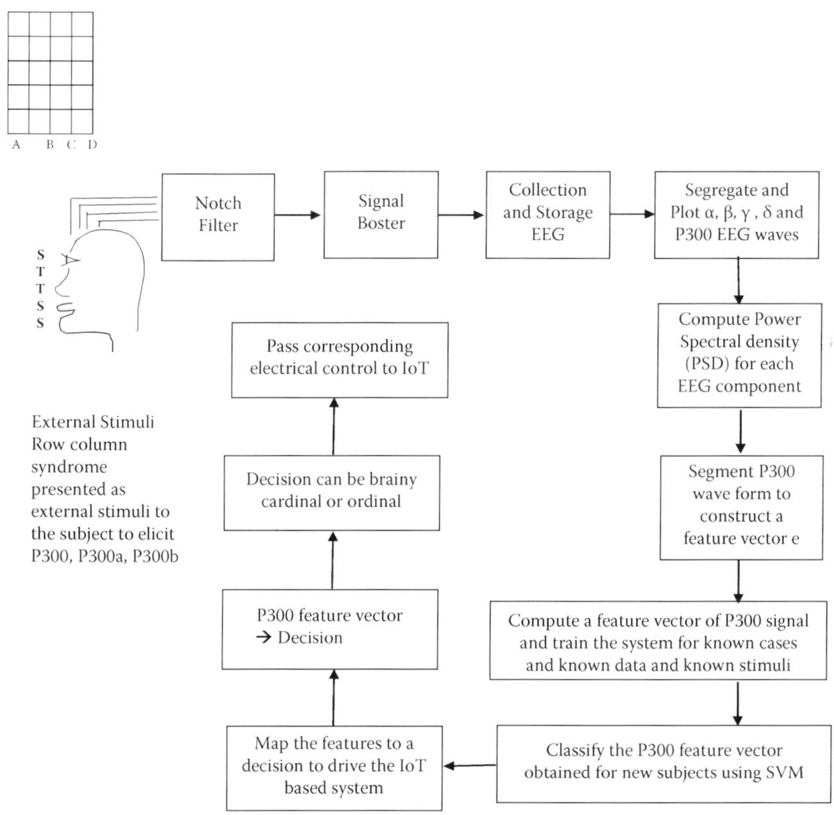

FIGURE 9.4 Process of BCI as a system to control IoT-based devices.

EEG and further subjected to PSD (power spectral density) analysis. Various unique combinations of the PSD and the characteristic vector obtained by quantizing the P300 wave are codified as feature vectors.

The feature vector is further classified and mapped to some intended physical action by the subject. The processes of classification and mapping is repeated for a sufficient amount of time to develop confidence. How some of the decisions are made based on the feature vector are listed for various scenarios.

9.3 P300 CLASSIFIER

No specific artifact correction or rejection procedure preceded classifier training and online classification because it was found that pursuing similar moving targets did not lead to strong EOG contamination of the data in pilot experiments.

For both classifier training and online classification, the EEG was filtered in a 1–10 Hz band with an FIR filter and decimated down to 20 Hz, and 1 s epochs starting from the stimulus onset were extracted. The amplitude values concatenated for all six EEG channels formed a feature vector. The number of target and non-target epochs for classifier training was 120 and 960, respectively. Classifier weights were obtained by Fisher discriminate analysis. During the main part of the experiment, the weights were applied to each epoch separately. In the single-trial mode, the attended ball was determined by the highest value of the classifier output. The same rule was used in the triple-trial mode and the test mode, with the only difference being that the classifier outputs were first averaged for each ball separately across the three and five trials, respectively. A block diagram depicting collection of a P300 and its segregation process from EEG data is given in Figure 9.5.

Examples of some of the feature vectors mapped to common decisions:

1. Binary Decision – On/off for lights, fans, or any electrical appliance. If the feature vector is mapped to an ordinal (0, 1, 2, 3…8) set, then based on the ordinal value, the degree of intensity of the appliance is set such as the intensity of light as per the ordinal value (Figure 9.6).
2. Ordinal value can be mapped to directional movement of the cursor, or wheelchair: (0, 1, 2, 3…8) → (N, NE, E, SE, S, SW,W, NW, N).
3. According to the ordinal mapping, the cursor on the screen can be modeled to any cardinal direction or the image on the screen can be panned in one of the cardinal directions or movements of the wheelchair in the cardinal direction.
4. Brainy Decisions → Alive or Awake. Based on the ratio of power spectral density, the condition of a patient or subject can be decided in terms of awake (non-anesthesia) or under the influence of anesthesia.
5. (P300 high and T) in oddball stimuli → Truth else lie. This is used in lie detection testing of any subject.

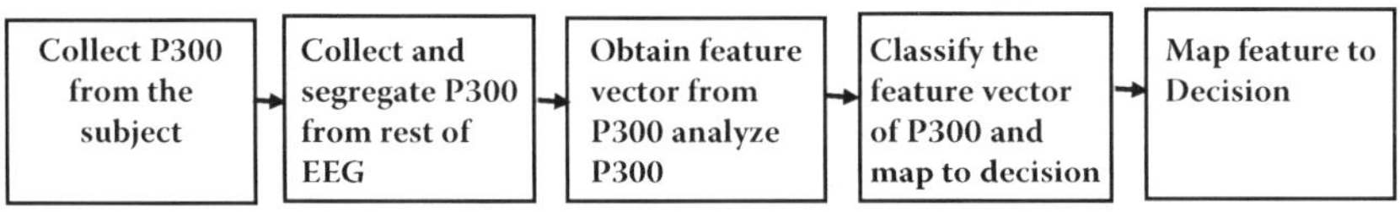

FIGURE 9.5 Process of collection of P300 and its segregation from EEG data.

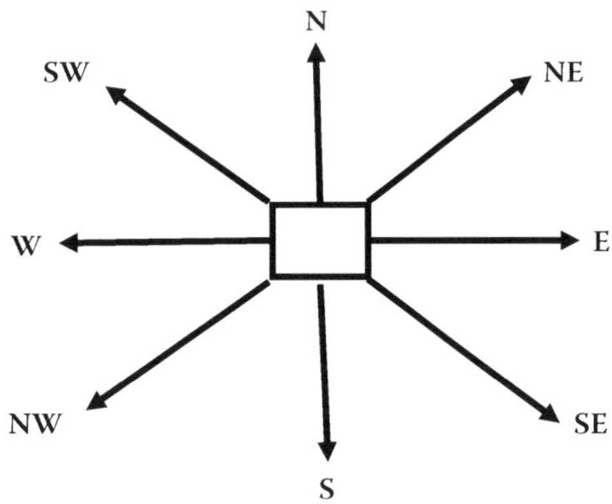

FIGURE 9.6 Binary decision.

9.3.1 ERP Analysis

Offline analysis was performed with MATLAB® (MathWorks, USA). The EEG and EOG channels were re-referenced to the average of the two earlobes and band-pass filtered using a second-order Butterworth filter in the forward and backward directions (for zero phase shift) in the range of 0.5–20 Hz, and epochs –0.2…0.6 s relative to the stimuli were extracted. Epochs with an amplitude exceeding ±50 μV in any channel were excluded from the analysis. The percentage of rejected epochs per participant and session never exceeded 11%. Visual screening of epochs extracted from non-filtered EEG confirmed that no significant artifacts escaped this procedure. Notably, strong artifacts from saccades were not common in our data, likely because pursuing the moving balls required only smooth-pursuit eye movement and small saccades. Blinking artifacts were also rare, likely because the stimulation periods were short.

The epochs were averaged separately for target and non-target stimuli per subject and session. For accuracy, in the case of the fourth session, the average values were computed separately for the first and second halves of the session, i.e., for the single-trial or triple-trial mode and for the test mode, respectively.

For the analysis of the N1 component, the PO7, PO8, O1, and O2 channels were averaged together. The N1 peak amplitude was estimated using this averaged signal as the maximum value in a 120–250 ms interval. The amplitude of the P300 peak was estimated as the maximum in the 250–500 ms interval at Pz. No baseline correction was used because filtering removed most of the slow variations in the signal. A slow negativity remained, however, in the beginning of the ERP waveforms. Averaging of longer epochs separately for different target positions within a stimulus sequence showed that this negativity started approximately 0.5 s before the first stimulus in the sequence and tended to grow if the target appeared later in the sequence (i.e., if the target-to-target interval was long). Therefore, the negativity may correspond to expectations of the target stimulus. No measures were taken to remove this component from the signal because the negativity seemed to disappear before the P300 wave reached its maximum.

9.4 P300 AS BCI

The ability of the human to communicate with each other plays a critical role in building a relationship with society and others. With the advent of modern logistics and necessities, communication between people has become richer and more complex than any other time of human history. Furthermore, as brain science and computer technologies mature, it is critical to have an ultimate interaction interface that will develop a direct communication between the user's brain and a computer; in other words, a BCI system that facilitates to build a real-time communication between a user and a computer system. The core purpose of a BCI is to detect brain activity in an EEG and communicate that activity to a computer or electronic device. A BCI allows a user to voluntarily send messages or control commands, bypassing the brain's natural output pathways. There have been different approaches for BCIs. A P300 BCI is a safe and non-invasive system, which requires the user to wear a small head cap carrying a set of electrical probes to detect brain P300 ERP. The P300 BCI has many potential advantages over many other input modes (Bayliss 2003).

9.5 ADVANTAGES OF A P300 FOR BCIS

There are some properties of a P300 that make it attractive for BCIs. Many applications include daily life uses: (1) the typical P300 BCI can be controlled with high accuracy; (2) the P300 BCI classifier offers fast response; (3) it may be used in gaming applications where an even shorter calibration can be used if classifier accuracy is not critical; (4) almost all healthy people and many severely paralyzed patients are able to use the P300 BCI; (5) unlike other BCIs such as the motor imagery-based BCI, no special training is needed to operate this BCI; and (6) a P300 BCI is non-invasive, calibration time is limited to few minutes, and it is effective for most users and more than 90% users feel comfortable with this system.

9.6 FUTURE USES OF A P300 BCI

There exist many future directions to improve the information throughput in P300 BCIs, which is also equally true for many other types of BCI systems. To uncover the applications of a P300 ERP to other modalities, an underlying physiological mechanism and brain response in each of the particular applications need to be carefully investigated. For example, a study to unfold more insight of the cognitive process showed that neurofeedback can be applied to augment the cognitive diagnosis. In order to increase the BCI accuracy, error correction mechanisms can be incorporated into the BCI system. It will also increase the user acceptability of a P300 BCI. Although improving information throughput of a BCI is of paramount importance, many other aspects of BCIs also demand substantial consideration. For example, future BCIs need to be faster, inexpensive, and easy to use. Fortunately, the BCI community comprises many other disciplines, such as engineering, cognitive and neuroscience, semantics, mathematics, psychology, clinical science, and software writing. Eventually, scientists and researchers from various avenues continuously help to find a universal platform for BCI development, utilizing available resources free for academic research. In particular, future expansion of BCI applications depends a lot on the thorough investigation of users' comfort in using BCIs. So different conditions should be well explored to find reasons behind why most users may or may not like a BCI system or paradigm. Many articles have introduced questionnaires and surveys to learn the comfort zone of the P300 BCI users. To promote the use of BCIs to the target users with new applications, records and studies of the human factors should be employed.

9.7 SUMMARY

This study investigated whether a P300 BCI stimuli can be presented on moving objects without a dramatic loss of classification accuracy. Participants successfully operated a game-like interface despite the attention and perceptional challenges raised by the movement of the stimulus positions. Moreover, the participants from both groups, practicing in either triple-trial (n = 6) or single-trial (n = 6) mode, maintained interest in their task across four sessions run on different days. The proposed BCI stimulus design, therefore, can be considered as a prospective basis for BCI games and might become a useful model for studying the effects of long-term BCI use in healthy people who are not motivated to use a BCI for communication or for control of robotics. The results also suggest that different stimulus items in the P300 BCI can be placed on separately moving parts of robotic devices.

Exercises

1. What is a brain computer interface (BCI)?
2. Draw a detailed diagram describing the functioning of a BCI using a P300 and label each of the components.
3. Draw a block diagram depicting various stages of signal processing used in a BCI.
4. How do you control an IoT device using a BCI?

5. Draw a process diagram of collection and delineation of a P300 from an EEG signal.
6. Give some examples of mapping of feature vectors extracted from an EEG signal to common decisions or operations.
7. What are the advantages of using a P300 for a BCI?
8. What are possible future uses of a P300 BCI?

REFERENCES

Bayliss, JD 2003, 'Use of the evoked potential P3 component for control in a virtual apartment,' *IEEE Transactions on Neural Systems and Rehabilitation Engineering*, vol. 11, pp. 113–116. doi:10.1109/TNSRE.2003.814438. PubMed: 12899249.

Congedo, M, Goyat, M, Tarrin, N, Ionescu, G, Varnet, L et al. 2011, 'Brain Invaders': A prototype of an open-source P300-based video game working with the OpenViBE platform,' in *Proceedings of the 5th International BCI Conference 2011*, Austria, Graz University of Technology, 22–24 September 2011, Graz: Verlag der Technischen Universität, pp. 280–283.

Donnerer, M & Steed, A 2010, 'Using a P300 brain-computer interface in an immersive virtual environment,' *Presence*, vol. 19, pp. 12–24. doi:10.1162/pres.19.1.12

Farwell, LA & Donchin, E 1988, 'Talking off the top of your head: Toward a mental prosthesis utilizing event-related brain potentials,' *Electroencephalography and Clinical Neurophysiology*, vol. 70, pp. 510–523. doi:10.1016/0013-4694(88)90149-6. PubMed: 2461285.

Guan, J, Chen, Y, Lin, J, Yuan, Y & Huang, M 2005, 'N2 components as features for brain computer interface,' in *Proceedings of the 2005 1st International Conference on Neural Interface and Control*, Wuhan, China, 26–28 May 2005, pp. 45–49.

Guger, C, Daban, S, Sellers, E, Holzner, C, Krausz, G et al. 2009, 'How many people are able to control a P300-based brain-computer interface (BCI)?,' *Neuroscience Letters*, vol. 462, pp. 94–98. doi:10.1016/j.neulet.2009.06.045. PubMed: 19545601.

Guo, F, Hong, B, Gao, X & Gao, S 2008, 'A brain-computer interface using motion-onset visual evoked potential,' *Journal of Neural Engineering*, vol. 5, pp. 477–485. doi:10.1088/1741-2560/5/4/011. PubMed: 19015582.

Hong, B, Guo, F, Liu, T, Gao, X & Gao, S 2009, 'N200-speller using motion-onset visual response,' *Clinical Neurophysiology*, vol. 120, pp. 1658–1666. doi:10.1016/j.clinph.2009.06.026. PubMed: 19640783.

Kaplan, AY, Lim, JJ, Jin, KS, Park, BW, Byeon, JG & Tarasova, SU 2005, 'Unconscious operant conditioning in the paradigm of brain-computer interface based on color perception,' *International Journal of Neuroscience*, vol. 115, pp. 781–802. doi:10.1080/00207450590881975. PubMed: 16019574.

Kaplan, AY, Shishkin, SL, Ganin, IP, Basyul, IA & Zhigalov, AY 2013, 'Adapting the P300 based brain-computer interface for gaming: A review,' *IEEE Transactions on Computational Intelligence and AI in Games*, vol. 5, pp. 141–149.

Liu, T, Goldberg, L, Gao, S & Hong, B 2010, 'An online brain-computer interface using non-flashing visual evoked potentials,' *Journal of Neural Engineering*, vol. 7, pp. 036003. doi:10.1088/1741-2560/7/3/036003. PubMed: 20404396.

Mak, JN, Arbel, Y, Minett, JW, McCane, LM, Yuksel, B et al. 2011, 'Optimizing the P300-based brain-computer interface: Current status, limitations and future directions,' *Journal of Neural Engineering*, vol. 8, pp. 025003. doi:10.1088/1741-2560/8/2/025003. PubMed: 21436525.

Plass-Oude Bos, D, Reuderink, B, van de Laar, B, Gürkök, H, Mühl, C et al. 2010, 'Brain-computer interfacing and games', in DSTan&A Nijholt (eds.)*Brain-Computer Interfaces*, pp. 149–178. Springer Verlag, London.

Rebsamen, B, Guan, C, Zhang, H, Wang, C, Teo, C et al. 2010, 'A brain controlled wheelchair to navigate in familiar environments,' *IEEE Transactions on Neural Systems and Rehabilitation Engineering*, vol. 18, pp. 590–598. doi:10.1109/TNSRE.2010.2049862. PubMed: 20460212.

Shishkin, SL, Ganin, IP & Kaplan, AY 2011, 'Event-related potentials in a moving matrix modification of the P300 brain-computer interface paradigm,' *Neuroscience Letters*, vol. 496, pp. 95–99. doi:10.1016/j.neulet.2011.03.089. PubMed: 21511006.

Wolpaw, JR 2007, 'Brain-computer interfaces as new brain output pathways,' *The Journal of Physiology*, vol. 579, pp. 613–619. doi:10.1113/jphysiol.2006.125948. PubMed: 17255164.

Wolpaw, JR, Birbaumer, N, McFarland, DJ, Pfurtscheller, G & Vaughan, TM 2002, 'Brain-computer interfaces for communication and control,' *Clinical Neurophysiology*, vol. 113, pp. 767–791. doi:10.1016/S1388-2457(02)00057-3. PubMed: 12048038.

Yuksel, B, Donnerer, M, Tompkin, J & Steed, A 2010, 'Using a P300 brain-computer interface in an immersive virtual environment,' in *Proceedings of the CHI 2010,* Atlanta, 10–15 April 2010, pp. 855–858.

Yuksel, BF, Donnerer, M, Tompkin, J & Steed, A 2011, 'Novel P300 BCI interfaces to directly select physical and virtual objects,' in *Proceedings of the 5th International BCI Conference2011*, Austria, Graz University of Technology, 22–24 September 2011, Graz: Verlag der Technischen Universität, pp. 288–291.

10 Designing an EEG Acquisition System

With the advent of VLSI technology, the ability to acquire, filter, and analyze low power and highly random signals has increased. Signal acquisition systems have become smaller, more accurate, portable, and more reliable. An EEG is a highly sought after signal acquisition system with a range of applications in neurological and psychiatry treatments. Yet this system is costly and often beyond the availability of a common patient. Therefore, designing an EEG system that is low in manufacturing cost and making it affordable for common patients yet robust enough to acquire EEG signals for critical study of neuropsychiatric analysis is important. This chapter gives a brief review of the current state of research in the field of EEG acquisition systems and signal processing of EEG signals and their applications to design a low-cost EEG system.

10.1 INTRODUCTION

According to scientific simulation and theoretical prediction, an adult human brain has 100 billion neurons and over 100 trillion neural connections or synapses that communicate with each other through electrical impulses. The systematic study of these electrical impulses passing through the synaptic connection between the neurons is known as electroencephalography (EEG). An EEG is a system that acquires and records the electrical activity of the brain (Matthews et al 2017).

The brain wave or EEG signal is the transient differential electrical potential between any two points on the scalp or between an electrode placed on the scalp and a reference electrode located elsewhere on the head. This potential difference oscillates rapidly at a frequency ranging from 0.1 to 50 Hz and gives rise to the characteristic "squiggly lines" that are referred to as "brain waves." Brain waves reflect change by becoming faster or slower in frequency or lower or higher in voltage, or perhaps some combination of these two responses (Kaplan & Sadock's 2015; Khan et al 2017).

Since the potential difference itself is extremely low in amplitude (10–100 μV), the electrodes used for acquiring the EEG signal must be sensitive enough to pick up and transmit the signal with minimum distortion. Krishnan et al. (2017) have compared EEG acquisition systems available in the market, while Pinegger et al. (2016) have compared different electrodes (gel-, water-, and dry-

DOI: 10.1201/9781003241386-10

based) available; both have independently concluded that different types of sensors and systems are suitable for different applications; there is no "one size fits all" EEG system available on the market that will be useful for different EEG applications.

Therefore, we propose the design of a versatile EEG acquisition system that is as accurate as a medical-grade system and at the same time, user friendly, robust, and cost effective compared to the available medical-grade EEG systems.

In the next section, we delve into the history of EEG systems and their evolution along with their increasing applications. Sections 10.2–10.4 discuss and puts forward the problem statement as a design challenge. In sections 10.5–10.7 we propose our indigenous design solution for a low-cost and robust EEG system.

10.2 REVIEW OF EEG APPLICATIONS

Since its inception in 1924, EEG systems have been used as tool for acquiring electrical brain waves for study of psychology, neuroscience, clinical, and psychiatric behavior. Due to extensive research in the field over the past decade or two, EEG acquisition is now more accurate and user friendly. As a result, its application has expanded to cover areas of research like neuromarketing, human factors, and social interactions.

In its initial stages, the application of an EEG was limited to psychiatrists and doctors who used it for detection of mental disorders like the study of epilepsy (Ullah et al 2018; Gajic et al 2014), psychiatric disorders (Mantri et al 2012; Al-Shargie et al 2016; Khosrowabadi 2017), sleep disorder analysis, learning disorders (Rogers et al 2018; Nami et al 2017), etc.

With the advancement of signal acquisition, electronic and signal processing EEG became more accessible to the general public along with its utilization in a wide variety of applications, all of which can be loosely categorized as brain machine interfaces (BMIs) or brain computer interfaces (BCIs). These applications begin with advanced, more accurate, and portable EEG acquisition systems (Uktveris & Jusas 2018; Luan et al 2014; Bhagawati & Chutia 2016; Jaganathan et al 2015; Xu et al 2004; Tian & Song 2016; Lakshmi et al 2014; Patil & Patil 2018), and then simple entertainment tasks like video games, media art, and music follow. We then come to applications based on control of computers (Lin et al 2014; Gomez-Gil et al 2011), prosthetics, wheelchairs (Jenita et al 2015), etc. Of late, an EEG is used for home automation (Sujatha & Ambica 2015; Alshbatat et al 2014; Anu et al 2016; Alhalaseh et al 2018; Alomari et al 2013) and other IoT-based services (Panigrahi et al 2020).

Lin et al. (Lin et al 2014), look at how commercially available EEG headsets compare to standardized tests and conclude that the data coming from the consumer headset is not only reliable but can also be used in everyday conditions and not just in controlled laboratory experimental conditions. The accuracy of such experiments is further supported by Gomez-Gill et al (2011). These researchers prove that not only EEG-based BCI and HMI applications are possible but also practical.

To implement any BCI application, the first and the most important thing to do is to acquire the EEG data accurately. Both Uktveris and Jusas (Uktveris & Jusas 2018) and Luan et al. (Luan et al 2014) propose a low-power, portable EEG acquisition system, but due to hardware filtering and constrictive EEG cap, their systems have inherent noise due to more hardware components, making it susceptible to EMI and EMC interference.

10.3 RESEARCH PROBLEMS

Following are some of the important problems encountered while designing an EEG acquisition system:

- Pickup, transmission, and amplification of EEG signal from scalp without introducing minimum noise in the system
- Reconstruction of EEG signal in the digital domain using ample number of samples from input analog signal
- Processing and feature extraction of digital data for further analysis and actuation-based applications
- Designing low-cost EEG acquisition systems with abundant channels capable of capturing accurate and reliable data

The gaps in research and design are clearly evident in research trends discussed in the next section. To address these problems, we aim to build the EEG acquisition-system using COTS (commercial off the shelf) hardware and in-house software to analyze and process the acquired data.

10.4 RESEARCH TRENDS

We carry out an explicit review of existing research literature to study the research trends. The manuscripts published between 2011 to date are considered for this review. The research papers published are categorized according to various problems they address and the number of papers are plotted in bar graph 1 (Figure 10.1). In bar graph 2 (Figure 10.2), the type of technology they adapt to design an EEG system is plotted.

10.5 PROPOSED SOLUTION

To design an EEG acquisition system, we will acquire the data using non-invasive, gold-plated Cu, and cup-shaped electrodes. The signal from the electrodes is fed to the instrumentation amplifier, and from there it goes to the microcontroller. Using the built-in ADC of the microcontroller, the signal is converted to a digital domain. The microcontroller is directly interfaced with MATLAB® for further digital filtration and feature extraction and analysis.

The problems encountered during our experiments and proposed improvements to overcome these issues are also discussed to achieve the final goal of making a versatile EEG acquisition system.

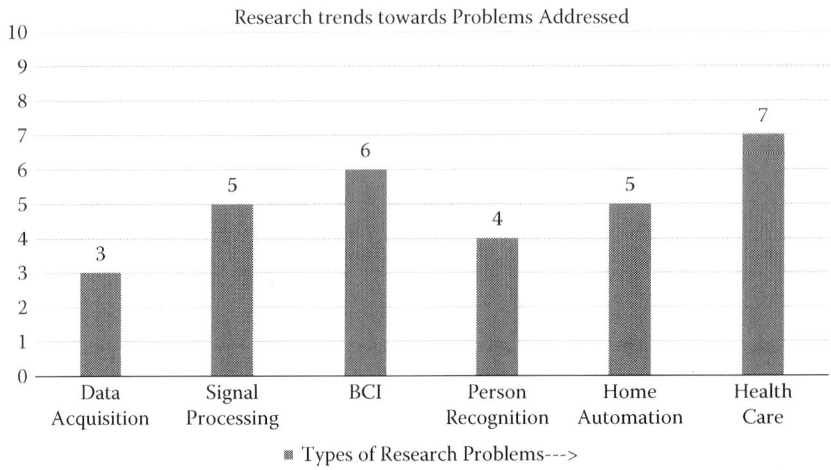

FIGURE 10.1 Research trends towards problems addressed.

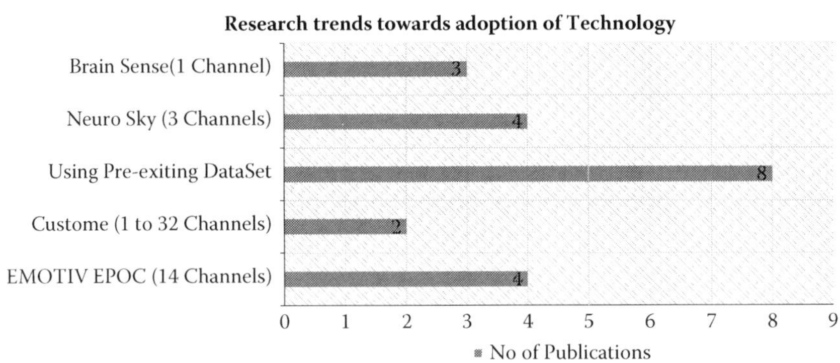

FIGURE 10.2 Research trends towards adoption of technology.

10.6 SYSTEM DESIGN

After careful examination of EEG signals and other medical-grade systems available on the market, the following design constraints to design the EEG acquisition system have been arrived at.

Design constraints:

- EEG voltage range: 10 μV to 100 μV
- EEG frequency range: 0.3 Hz to 60 Hz
- Max variation of input signal per unit time: 50 μV
- Sampling rate: 256 to 1k SPS

The subsequent sections talk about the step-by-step design of each component in the acquisition system.

10.6.1 Block Diagram

The block diagram (Figure 10.3) gives an overview of the proposed system to acquire an EEG signal. The signal acquired is first pre-processed. The processing of an EEG signal and its subsequent visualization and interpretation is performed through MATLAB programs developed to identify different artifacts present in the EEG signal.

10.6.2 Electrodes

The electrodes used for our system are a dry, non-invasive type that are applied with the help of a conductive paste of saline solution. The electrodes have the following specifications:

- Gold-plated copper
- Dimensions – Diameter of cup: 10 mm
- Height of cup: 3.5 mm
- 2-mm hole in the center
- 1.5-mm DIN42802 female touch-proof connector
- Form factor: cup shaped

10.6.3 Electrode Placement

The electrodes are placed based on the international 10–20 system, which measures the distance between identifiable landmarks on the head and then locates electrode positions at 10% or 20% of that distance in an anterior–posterior or transverse direction. Electrodes are then designated by an uppercase letter denoting the brain region beneath that electrode and a number, with odd numbers used for the left hemisphere and even numbers signifying the right hemisphere (the subscript Z denotes midline electrodes). For example, the O2 electrode is placed over the right occipital region, and the P3 lead is found over the left parietal area (Figure 10.4).

10.6.4 Electrode Cap

The electrode cap selected is of standard size made of an elastic material (as opposed to a 3D-printed cap) to ensure a snug fit on heads of all shapes and sizes to maintain proper contact between the electrodes and the scalp.

The cap further has cups to hold up to 32 electrodes, giving the user the freedom to place electrodes where most significant data is picked up based on the application when using less than 32 electrodes (Figure 10.5).

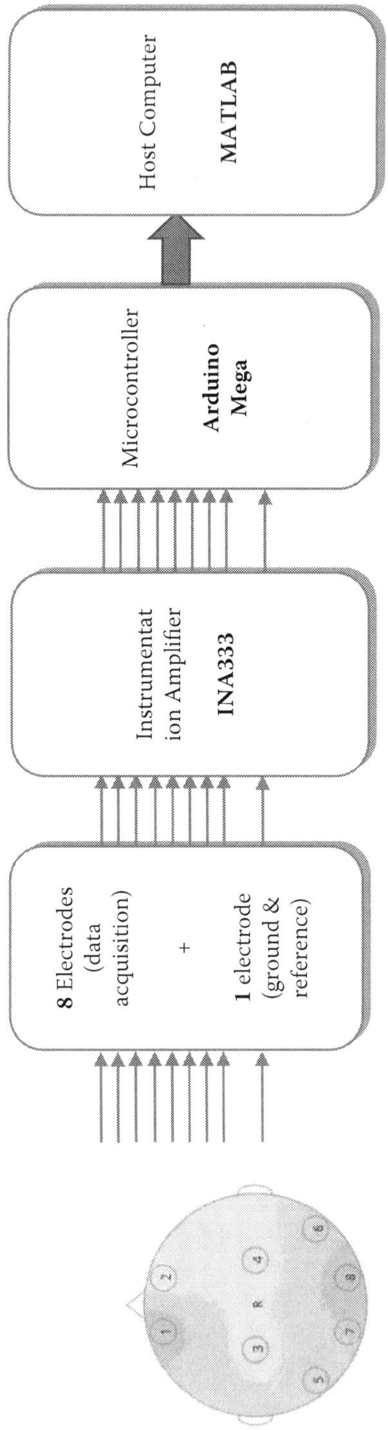

FIGURE 10.3 The block diagram depicts the process for obtaining an EEG signal.

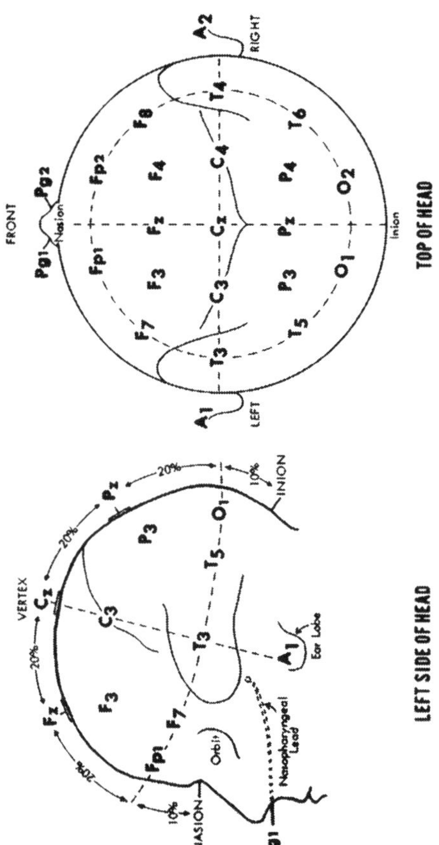

FIGURE 10.4 International 10–20 electrode placement system. (Courtesy Kaplan & Sadock's 2015.)

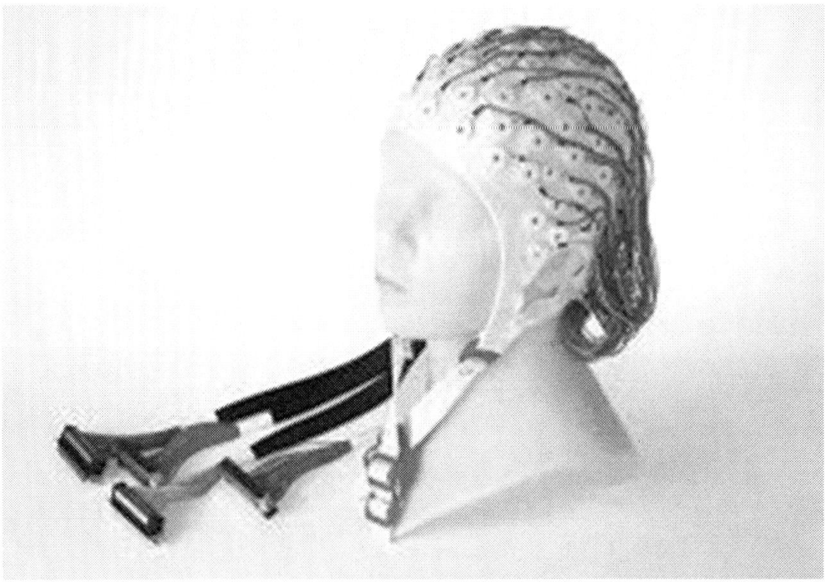

FIGURE 10.5 Electrode cap.

10.6.5 Instrumentation Amplifier

The instrumentation amplifier best suited for this application is an INA333 due to its low-input offset voltage (25 μV), high CMRR (100 dB), and high gain (1,000).

INA118 was a viable alternative, but was rejected due to its high-input offset voltage (50 μV), which is comparable to the EEG signal itself.

10.6.6 Microcontroller

The microcontroller used for this application is Arduino Mega. With a clock speed of 16 MHz, operating voltage of 5 V, and a 10-bit in-built ADC, the Mega can directly take analog input from the instrumentation amplifier and give digital data to the host computer. Arduino also provides a direct interface with MATLAB, which makes signal filtration and further processing much easier.

The Arduino Due has better specifications but was rejected because of its low operating voltage of 3.3 V and lack of online support libraries.

Raspberry Pie was rejected due to lack of GPIO ports and interface capabilities with the future use of an analog front end.

10.6.7 Bill of Materials Required to Assemble a EEG Acquisition System

A bill of materials (BOM) is a list of the raw materials, sub-assemblies, intermediate assemblies, sub-components, parts, and the quantities of each needed to manufacture an end product. A BOM may be used for communication between manufacturing partners or confined to a single manufacturing plant. A bill of materials is often tied to a production order whose issuance may generate reservations for components in the bill of materials that are in stock and requisitions for components that are not in stock.

In electronics, the BOM represents the list of components used on the printed wiring board or printed circuit board. Once the design of the circuit is completed, the BOM list is passed on to the PCB layout engineer as well as the component engineer, who will procure the components required for the design. Given below is the BOM (Table 10.1) for the design and assembly of an EEG acquisition system.

10.7 TESTING AND OBSERVATIONS

The Arduino IDE is neither capable of proper reconstruction and representation of the incoming signal nor is it capable of further processing; hence, Arduino is interfaced to MATLAB, which is then used to plot a real-time frequency domain and time domain spectrum of the incoming EEG signal.

Figure 10.7 shows the same experiment performed as in Figure 10.6. Subplot 1 shows the real-time RAW EEG signal amplified 101 times, whereas subplot 2 shows the real-time frequency plot (FFT). In FFT, the peaks show a concentration of a signal at that particular frequency.

It is clearly observed and inferred that acquiring data in MATLAB is the better option.

Figure 10.9 shows the comparison of saccade, fix, and blink data. Subplot 1 shows the data from our system, while subplot 2 shows the data from the medical-grade system. This is similar for subplots 3 and 4.

TABLE 10.1
Bill of materials

Sl No.	Component	Amount	Cost (INR)
1	EEG cap	1	2,500
2	EEG electrodes	9	3,009
3	EEG paste	228 g	1,500
4	Instrumentation amplifier INA333	9	4,613
5	Active and passive elements + amplifiers for filter design	Requirement based	500
6	Arduino Mega 2560 REV3	1	699
7	Fabrication cost of PCB	Need based	10,000
Total		INR 12,821 (components) + 10,000 (fabrication) = INR 22,821	

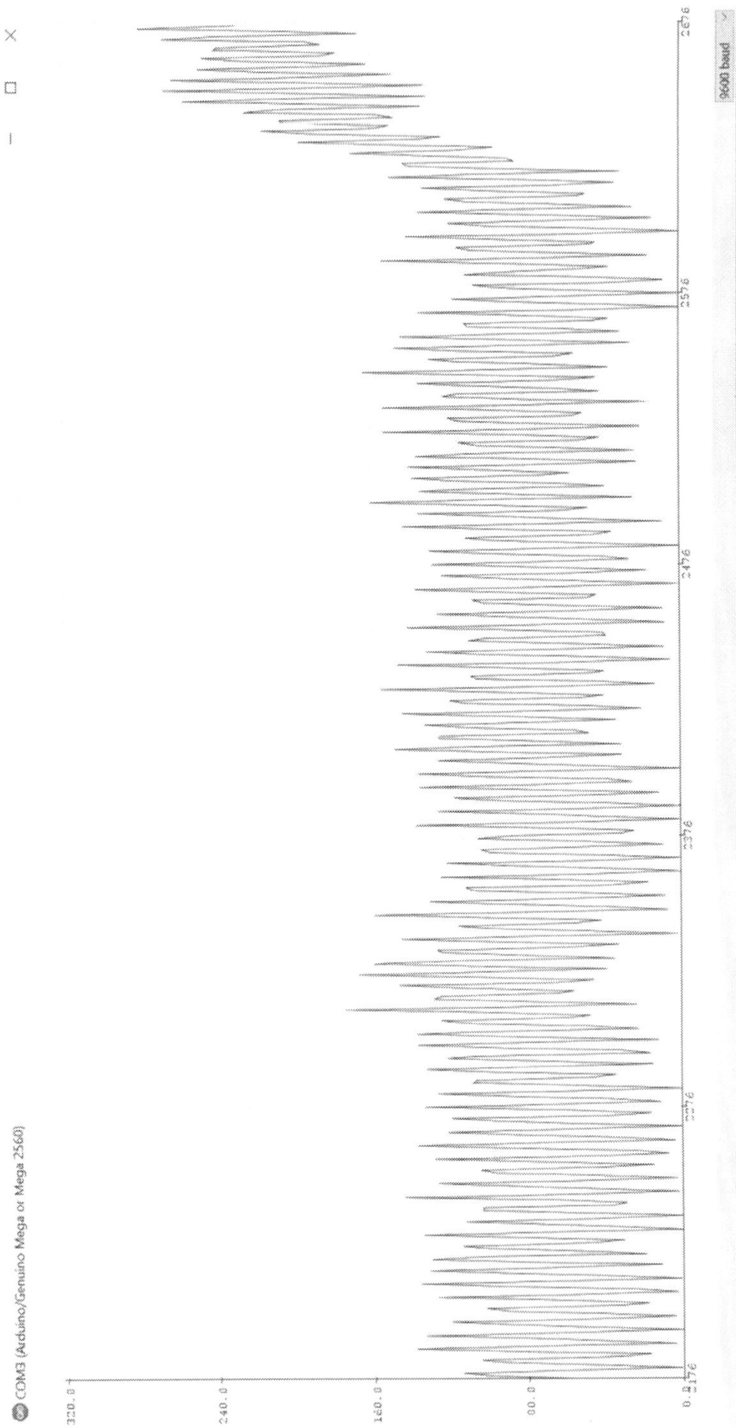

FIGURE 10.6 Data acquisition in MATLAB interfaced with Arduino.

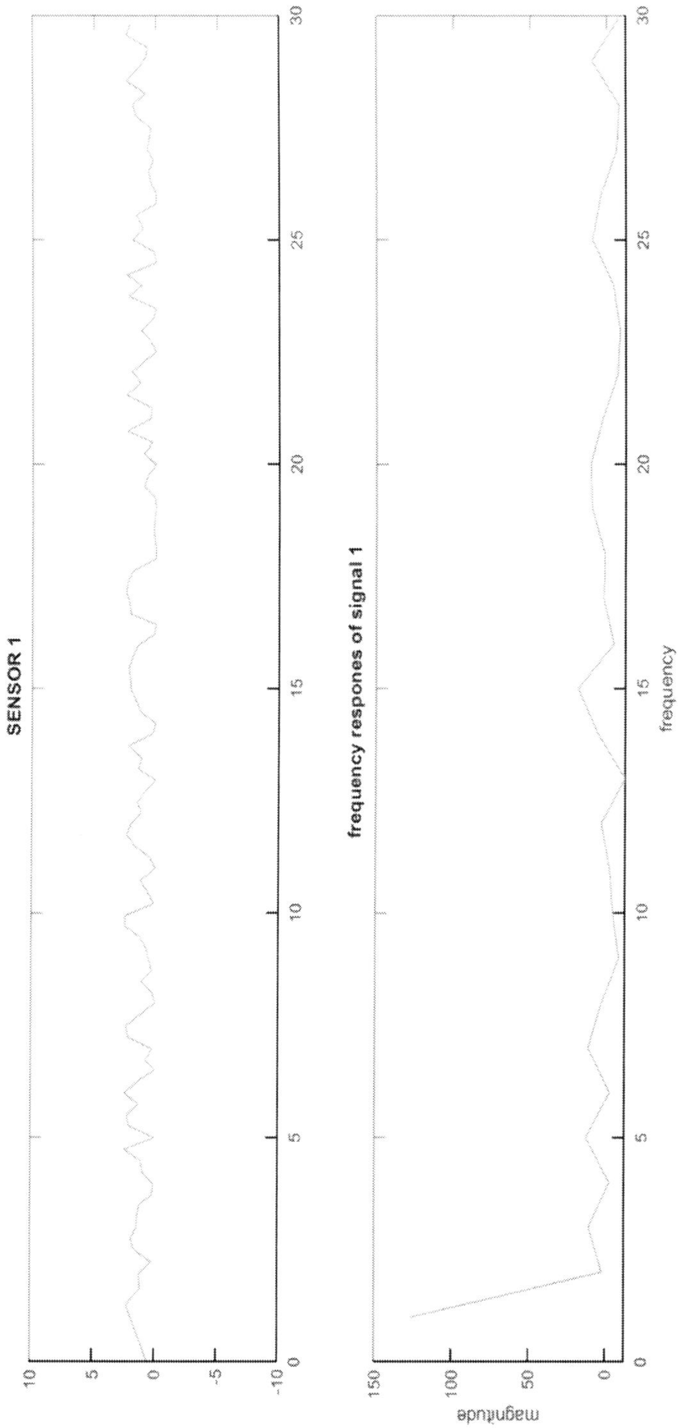

FIGURE 10.7 Shows the acquired EEG data represented in Arduino IDE at a lower baud rate. The single-channel output is connected to analog port A0 of the Arduino.

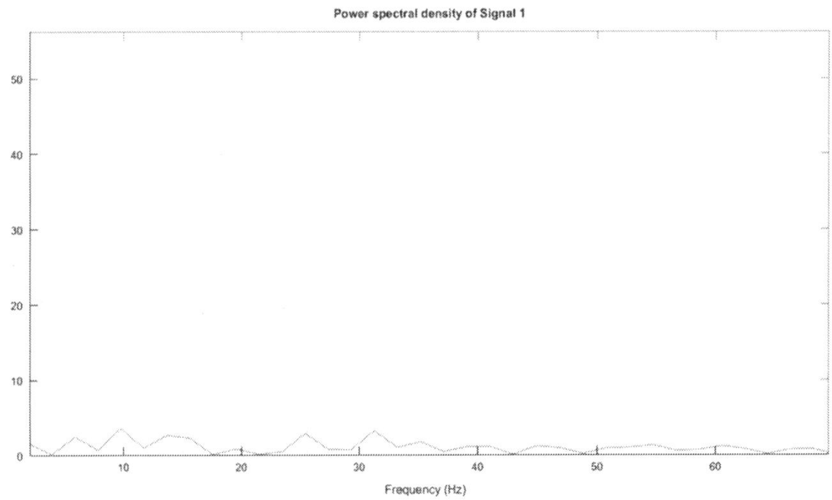

FIGURE 10.8 Power spectral density of data acquired from a single sensor coming from an instrumentation amplifier with a gain of 101.

It is evident from the figure that our proposed system captures the correct data, as all peaks match between both signals. The drawback here is the low sampling rate because the reconstructed signal does not have as much detail as is required for complex analysis – this can be seen when comparing subplots 3 and 4.

The maximum rate at which the data is captured is about 5 Hz.

To overcome the drawback, we tried to increase the baud rate of Arduino.

Figure 10.10 clearly sees an improvement in the reconstruction of the acquired signal when compared to the output seen in Figure 10.6 at a lower baud rate.

Trying to achieve such high baud rates in the interface with MATLAB is difficult due to the constraints of the Arduino toolbox. As a result, the next experiment is carried out with the help of serial transmission of data from Arduino to MATLAB.

As observed in Figure 10.10, the reconstruction of data is much better when compared to the data acquired in Figure 10.6. But even after taking the baud rate up to 115,200, the rate at which data is captured is still about 10 Hz.

10.8 RESULTS AND DISCUSSION

As observed in the previous section, the use of MATLAB over Arduino IDE is justified because of better data representation and the availability of tools to further process and filter the incoming data.

Arduino Mega is used instead of Arduino Due because the output waveforms start getting clipped off due to the limited power supplied by Due because of the instrumentation amplifier.

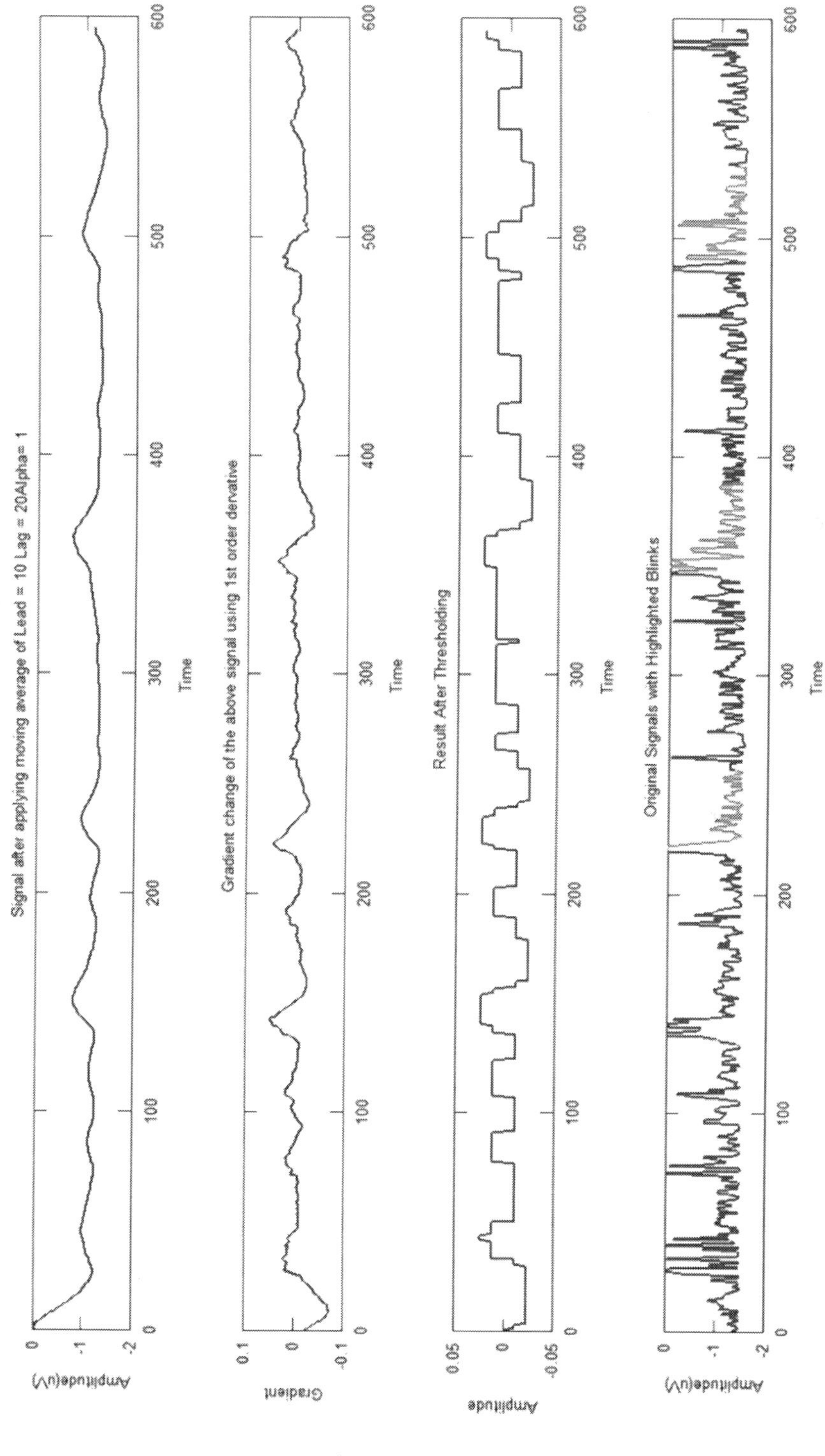

FIGURE 10.9 Comparison of data acquired from a medical-grade system and our proposed system.

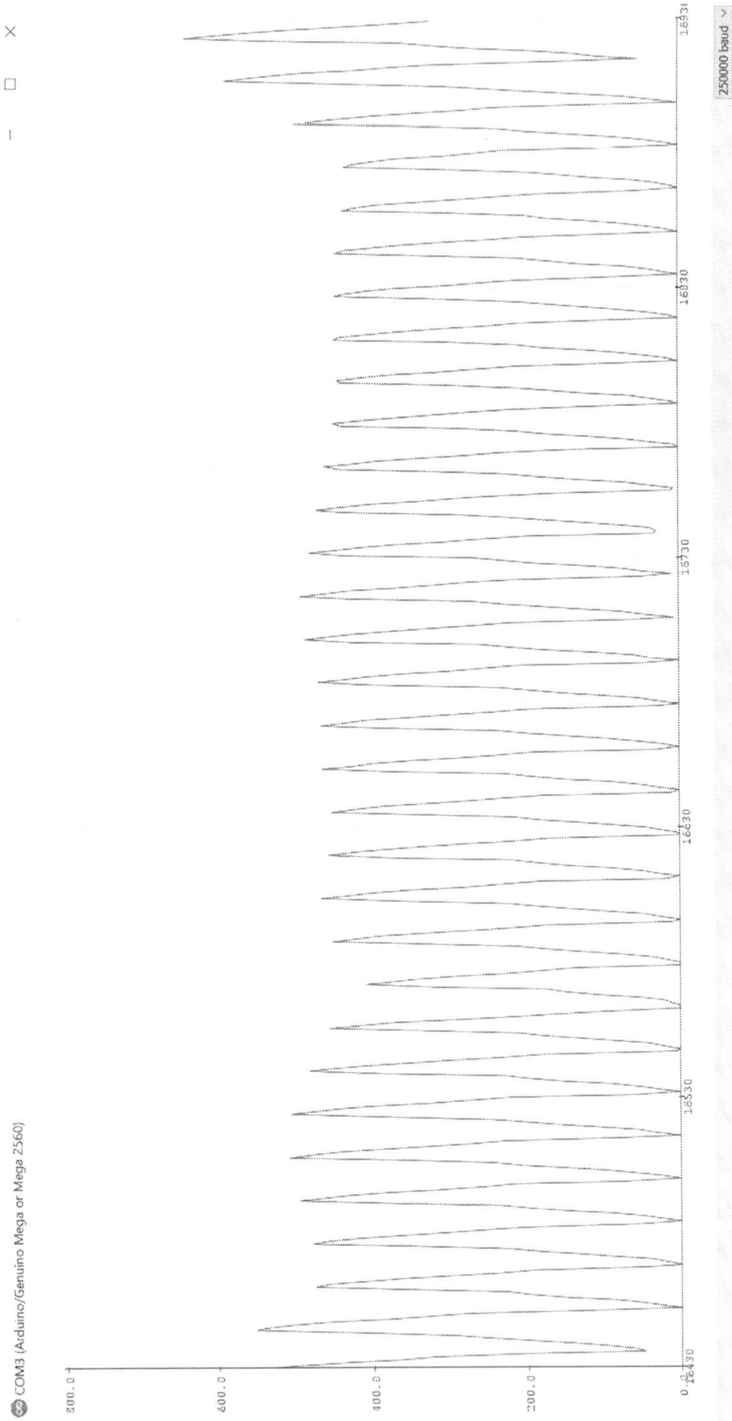

FIGURE 10.10 Data acquisition in Arduino IDE at 250,000 baud rate.

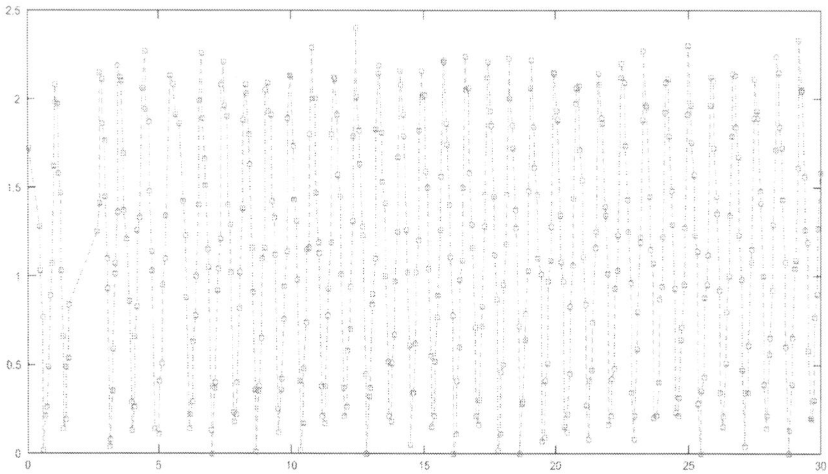

FIGURE 10.11 Serial transmission of data from Arduino IDE to MATLAB at 115,200 baud rate.

The power spectral density in Figure 10.8 shows peaks in the EEG data that correspond to alpha, beta, gamma, theta, and delta waves, which in addition to the comparison in Figure 10.9, proves the accuracy of our proposed system.

The only drawback in the current system is the low sampling rate because the signal is not being reconstructed properly, which in turn results in the loss of information . According to the Nyquist sampling theorem, considering a practical system with a maximum usable frequency of 50 Hz, the minimum sampling rate should be 125 Hz. This can only be achieved using an analog front end (suggested ADS1299) chip.

10.9 CONCLUSION

From the above design, the following can be concluded:

The proposed system captures accurate EEG signal despite using low cost electronic systems in designing the overall system, making it a low cost instrument for capturing EEG. In order to improve the robustness of the signal captured, an ADC (preferably ADS1299) must be introduced between the instrumentation amplifier and the microcontroller. To increase the number of EEG signal channels to be captured through the proposed system more ADS1299 to be daisy-chained.It will also make the system modular and robust where more input channels can be added on demand based on the needs of the user (Figure 10.11).

Exercises

1. What are the important design criteria encountered in designing an EEG acquisition system?

2. State some of the design constraints in designing an EEG acquisition system.
3. Give a block diagram with various components used in the design of an EEG system.
4. What are different electrode placement schemes used in an EEG acquisition system?
5. Describe different active, passive, and software components required in designing an EEG system.
6. Give a brief review of research applications of EEGs.
7. Give a brief note on some of the research problems in EEG system designs.
8. Give a brief note on different research uses of EEGs.
9. Compare and contrast the specification of EEG data, acquisition system, and processing and requirements between a research grade and medical-grade EEG system.
10. Give a bill of materials required to assemble an EEG acquisition system.

REFERENCES

Alhalaseh, K, Migdadi, H, Alhalaseh, R & Al-Gara, M 2018, 'Home automation application using EEG sensor,' in *Proceedings of 98th The IRES International Conference*, Antalya, Turkey, 21–22 January.

Alomari, MH, Samaha, A & AlKamha, K 2013, 'Automated classification of L/R hand movement EEG signals using advanced feature extraction and machine learning,' *(IJACSA) International Journal of Advanced Computer Science and Applications*, vol. 4, no. 6, pp. 207–212.

Al-Shargie, F, Tang, TB, Badruddin, N & Kiguchi, M 2016, 'Mental stress quantification using EEG signals,' *International Conference for Innovation in Biomedical Engineering and Life Sciences*, vol. 56, pp. 15–19, Research Gate Publication.

Alshbatat, AIN, Vial, PJ, Premaratne, P & Tran, LC 2014 September, 'EEG-based brain-computer interface for automating home appliances,' *Journal of Computers*, vol. 9, no. 9, pp. 2159–2166.

Anu, KE, Joseph, J, Narayanan, S, George, S & Joy, MM 2016 March, 'Non invasive electroencephalograph control for smart home automation,' *International Journal of Advanced Research in Electrical, Electronics and Instrumentation Engineering*, vol. 5, no. 3, pp. 115–121.

Bhagawati, AJ & Chutia, R 2016 January, 'Design of single channel portable eeg signal acquisition system for brain computer interface application,' *International Journal of Biomedical Engineering and Science (IJBES)*, vol. 3, no. 1, pp. 37–44.

Gajic, D, Djurovic, Z, Gennaro, SD & Gustafsson, F 2014, 'Classification of EEG signals for detection of epileptic seizures based on wavelets and statistical pattern recognition,' *Biomedical Engineering: Applications, Basis and Communications*, vol. 26, no. 2, pp. 1450021-1–1450021-13.

Gomez-Gil, J, San-Jose-Gonzalez, I, Nicolas-Alonso, LF & Alonso-Garcia, S 2011, 'Steering a tractor by means of an EMG-based human-machine interface,' *MDPI Sensors*, vol. 11, no. 7, pp. 7110–7126. ISSN 1424-8220.

Jaganathan, C, Amudhavalli, A, Janani, T, Dhanalakshmi, M & Madian, N 2015 April, 'Automated algorithm for extracting α, β, δ, θ of a human EEG,' *International Journal of Science, Engineering and Technology Research (IJSETR)*, vol. 4, no. 4.

Jenita, B, Rani, A & Umamakeswari, A 2015 May, 'Electroencephalogram-based brain controlled robotic wheelchair,' *Indian Journal of Science and Technology*, vol. 8, no. S9, pp. 188–197.

Khan, ZH, Hussain, N & Tiwana, MI 2017, 'Classification of EEG signals for wrist and grip movements using echo state network,' *Biomedical Research*, vol. 28, no. 3, pp. 1095–1102.

Khosrowabadi, R 2017, 'Stress and perception of emotional stimuli: Long-term stress rewiring the brain,' *Basic and Clinical Neuroscience*, vol. 9, no. 2, pp. 107–120.

Krishnan, NM, Mariappan, M, Muthukaruppan, K, Hijazi, MHA & Kitt, WW 2017, 'Electroencephalography (EEG) based control in assistive mobile robots: A review,' *IOP Conference Series: Materials Science and Engineering*, vol. 121, no. 1.

Lakshmi, MR, Dr. Prasad, TV & Dr. Prakash, VC 2014 January, 'Survey on EEG signal processing methods,' *International Journal of Advanced Research in Computer Science and Software Engineering*, vol. 4, no. 1, pp. 84–91.

Lin, Y-P, Wang, Y & Jung, T-P 2014, 'Assessing the feasibility of online SSVEP decoding in human walking using a consumer EEG headset,' *Journal of NeuroEngineering and Rehabilitation*, vol. 11, no. 1, 119.

Luan, B, Sun, M & Jia, W 2014, 'Portable amplifier design for a novel EEG monitor in point-of-care applications,' in , 16–18 March 2012, Philadelphia, PA, USA. doi: 10.1109/NEBC.2012.6207127 Proceedings of the IEEE Annual Northeast Bioengineering Conference

Mantri, S, Patil, V & Mitkar, R 2012 October, 'EEG based emotional distress analysis – A survey,' *International Journal of Engineering Research and Development*, vol. 4, no. 6, pp. 24–28.

Matthews, G, Reinerman-Jones, L, Abich, J IV & Kustubayeva, A 2017, 'Metrics for individual differences in EEG response to cognitive workload: Optimizing performance prediction,' *Personality and Individual Differences*, vol. 118, pp. 22–28.

Nami, M, Mehrabi, S & Derman, S 2017, 'Employing neural network methods to label sleep EEG micro-arousals in obstructive sleep apnea syndrome,' *Journal of Advanced Medical Sciences and Applied Technologies*, vol. 3, no. 4, pp. 221–226.

Panigrahi, N et al. 2020, 'Design of a robust EEG acquisition system for IoT applications,' *Advances in Science, Technology and Engineering Systems*, vol. 5, no. 2, pp. 119–129.

Patil, NR & Patil, SN 2018 March–April, 'Review: Wavelet transform based electroencephalogram methods,' *International Journal of Trend in Scientific Research and Development (IJTSRD)*, vol. 2, no. 3, pp. 1776–1779.

Pinegger, A, Wriessnegger, SC, Faller, J & Müller-Putz, GR 2016, 'Evaluation of different EEG acquisition systems concerning their suitability for building a brain–Computer interface: Case studies,' *Frontiers in Neuroscience*, vol. 10, Article 441.

Rogers, JM, Bechara, J & Johnstone, SJ 2018, 'Acute EEG patterns associated with transient ischemic attack,' *Clinical EEG and Neuroscience*, vol. 50, no. 3, pp. 196–204.

Sadock, BJ, Sadock, VA & Ruiz, P 2015, *Kaplan & Sadock's Synopsis of Psychiatry – Behavioral Sciences – Clinical Psychiatry*, Lippincott Williams & Wilkins, Philadelphia.

Sujatha, B & Ambica, G 2015 December, 'EEG based brain computer interface for controlling home appliances,' *International Research Journal of Engineering and Technology (IRJET)*, vol. 2, no. 09, pp. 580–585.

Tian, J & Song, W 2016 October–December, 'LabVIEW for EEG signal processing,' *Saudi Journal of Engineering and Technology*, vol. 1, no. 4, pp. 190–193.

Uktveris, T & Jusas, V 2018, 'Development of a modular board for EEG signal acquisition,' *MDPI Sensors*, vol. 18, no. 7, 2140. doi: 10.3390/s18072140.

Ullah, I, Hussain, M, Qazi, E-U-H & Aboalsamh, H 'An automated system for epilepsy detection using EEG brain signals based on deep learning approach,' *International Journal- Expert Systems with Applications*, vol. 107, pp. 61–71.

Xu, W, Guan, C, Siong, CE, Ranganatha, S, Thulasidas, M. & Wu, J 2004, 'High accuracy classification of EEG signal,' in *Proceedings of the* , vol. 2, pp. 391–394. doi: 10.1109/ICPR.2004.1334229. 17th International Conference on Pattern Recognition (ICPR'04) Cambridge, UK.

11 A Method to Localize the Pupil of the Eye for Point of Gaze Estimation

OVERVIEW

Estimating a gaze point through localization of the pupil in the image of the eye through optical eye-tracking during opto-ocular motion of the eye possesses many challenges. This chapter discusses a method to estimate the point of gaze on a digital screen using a non-intrusive eye tracking technique. In this method, a modified web camera is used to obtain the center of the pupil and is processed further to obtain the point of gaze.

11.1 INTRODUCTION

The estimation of the point of a gaze in a scene presented in a digital screen has many applications, such as fatigue detection and attention tracking. Some popular applications of eye tracking through gaze estimation are depicted in Figure 11.1. For estimation of point of gaze, it is required to identify the visual focus of a person within a scene. This is known as eye fix or point of fixation. Finding the point of gaze involves tracking different features of human eyes. Various methods are available for eye tracking. Some of them use special contact lenses (Robinson 1963) and some others use electrical potential measurement (Bulling 2011). The optical tracking of eyes is a non-intrusive tracking technique that uses a sequence of image frames of eyes recorded using video capturing devices. This technique is popularly known as video oculography (VOG). Different techniques used in VOG for the purpose of eye tracking are pupil-corneal reflection vectors or Purkinje images (Crane & Steele 1985) and pupil-eye corner vectors (Zhu & Yang 2012).

All of these techniques successfully work only if two or more features of the eyes are detected accurately. This increases the computational complexity, thereby limiting the speed of eye tracking systems. Some commercial eye tracking equipment available on the market are Eyelink-1000, SMI, and Tobii glasses. The cost of these systems is quite high and therefore can be used only for research purposes. In this article, a low-cost system is proposed that uses a modified web camera to obtain fixation points of subjects within a scene using

DOI: 10.1201/9781003241386-11

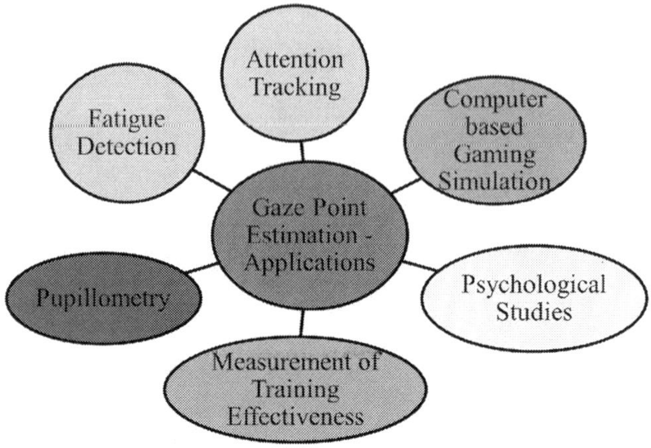

FIGURE 11.1 Applications of gaze point estimation.

the center of the pupil. The system is capable of generating 25–30 frames per second, which is sufficient to compute the position and size of the pupil in the pixels. Eye tracking and gaze position estimation have many applications.

11.2 PREVIOUS RESEARCH ON GAZE ESTIMATION

In 1981, Levine (1981), in his research article, first reported the application of eye tracking for an eye-controlled computer. Hutchinson and White (Duchowski 2002) have reported eye gaze as an input for human-computer interaction. A survey of research literature on eye-tracking applications was reported by Duchowski (Wang & Sung 2002) and Wang (Yoo & Chung 2005) in 2002. Different eye-tracking algorithms, applications, and methods were reported (Sugioka et al 1996; Lee et al 2010). Corcoran et al. (2012) have reported many interesting applications of real-time eye gaze tracking for gaming designs and consumer electronics systems.

Eye tracking can be done using methods such as 2D regression and 3D modeling of the eye. The 3D modeling methods implement a geometric model of the eye to estimate the point of intersection of visual axis and the scene. These systems typically use a single camera and were studied by Meyer et al. (2006), Guestrin and Eizenman (Guestrin & Eizenman 2006), and Henessey et al. (Hennessey et al 2006). Guestrin and Eizenman (Guestrin & Eizenman 2006) proposed that the number of cameras and light sources be increased, to reduce the number of parameters to be determined during calibration. This proposal was validated by the works of Shih (Lai et al 2015), Ohno (Ohno & Mukawa 2004), Beymer (Beymer & Flickner 2003), and Zhu (Zhu & Ji 2007), whose models utilize two or more cameras. However, these models might require multiple cameras or complex mathematical models for estimation of the center of the cornea and to estimate the visual axis. The other popular method is a 2D regression technique. In this method, the pupil – glint vector is mapped to the gaze coordinates by using a mapping function. This mapping function can be resolved using polynomial regression or artificial neural networks. Blignaut (2013) and Cherif et al. (2002) describe various methods used for calibration and deducing mapping functions using a regression technique. Chuang (Jian-nan et al 2009) propose systems that implement artificial neural networks for determining the mapping function used for translating pupil – glint vector to gaze points. All of these regression techniques depend on accurate detection of two or more features of the eye for accurate tracking. Corcoran et al. (2012) proposed a system that detects human face in an image followed by detection of eyes and estimate the center of the pupil from the image. Due to this, the image of the eye should be processed multiple times to detect all the required features. The accuracy of the system depends on accurate identification of these features. This uses a considerable amount of computational effort, leading to slow performance of the system. Through this, we propose a system that uses only a single feature, the center of the pupil, to estimate the point of gaze.

The first step of obtaining the point of gaze is to obtain coordinates of the center of the pupil from snapshots of the eye of a subject. There are two popular ways of performing that in the snapshots: (1) passive imaging and (2) active imaging (Hansen & Dan 2010; Lifeng & Yuyanchao 2009).

Passive imaging uses visible light available in the surroundings to capture images of the eyes, as depicted in Figure 11.2. These images are processed to detect various features of the eyes such as eye corners and pupil. However, the pupil cannot be identified accurately as there is little contrast between the pupil and the iris. This imaging is also affected by external lighting conditions, leading to errors in detection of features. Moreover, in the passive imaging process, various objects in the surroundings are also reflected on the surface of the eye, which adds additional artifacts. These reflections are to be eliminated during the processing stages of the image.

Active imaging uses an illumination source along with the imaging device. If the illumination source emits light in the visible spectrum, it causes discomfort to the user and limits the duration for which the experiment can be conducted. Also, there will be no contrast between the pupil and iris, leading to less accuracy in the detection of the center of the pupil.

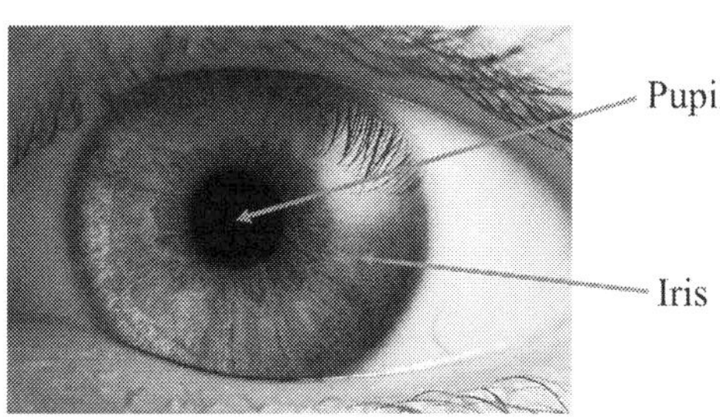

FIGURE 11.2 Image of eye captured using passive imaging.

The other type of active imaging source uses IR illumination. IR light is invisible to human eyes and hence does not cause any discomfort to the user. Another advantage is that it produces a high contrast between the iris and the pupil. This is because of the presence of melanin in the iris. Melanin is a chromophore that is responsible for the dark color of the iris. Melanin absorbs visible light and hence appears dark in visible light. However, absorption of light that falls in the near IR wavelength by melanin is negligible. Hence, it appears as a gray color in IR light. The pupil, however, is a lens made up of transparent liquid and will let IR light pass through it. The pupil might appear in two different ways in IR light based on the position of the illumination source. If the source is coaxial to the optical axis of the eye, the IR light gets reflected from the retina and illuminates the pupil, leading to a bright pupil effect as depicted in Figure 11.3(a). If the illumination source is offset from the optical path, the retro reflection from the retina is directed away from the camera, causing a dark pupil effect as depicted in Figure 11.3(b). The bright pupil effect is difficult to obtain due to the requirement that the illumination source has to be coaxial to the optical path. This requires a specialized IR illumination source. On the other hand, the dark pupil effect can be produced easily and hence it is a widely used technique for eye tracking.

11.2.1 Detection of the Pupil

The main feature required for any eye tracker is to detect the (x, y) coordinates of the center of the pupil. However, to identify the relative motion of the pupil, at least one other feature that stays fixed during eye movements is required. This feature can be an eye corner or a glint formed by the IR illumination source. The vector of pupil-glint or pupil-eye corner can be used to obtain the point of regard on a screen, allowing slight freedom in movement of the user's head. However, if the head pose of the viewer is stabilized, (x, y) coordinates of the center of the pupil alone is sufficient to obtain the eye fix. This reduces the computational complexity required to identify other features of the eye, such as glints and eye corners.

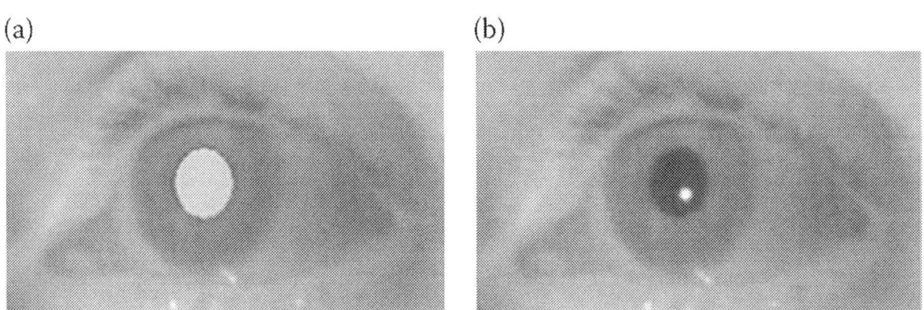

FIGURE 11.3 (a) Bright pupil effect; (b) Dark pupil effect.

The detection of the location of the pupil is a key feature of any eye-tracking mechanism. The accuracy of the system largely depends on accurate detection of the center of the pupil for all positions of the eyes. The detection of the pupil is easier when using a bright or dark pupil effect (refer Figure 11.3(b)). For simplicity, the discussion is limited to the dark pupil effect. The first step is to acquire an image of the eye using an IR camera. The dark regions in this frame consist of eyelashes, a part of eyebrow, and the pupil. Of all these dark regions, the pupil has a well-defined shape and is the largest connected component in the entire image. The second step is to obtain a binary image that consists of dark regions only. This can be achieved by applying an intensity threshold transformation to the image. A threshold value is chosen that represents the value of intensity of color in each pixel that is to be considered as dark. If all three values of any pixel i.e., R, G, and B, are less than the threshold value, then that pixel is considered as dark. Thus, all the pixels with RGB values above the threshold are painted in white and all the pixels with RGB values less than or equal to the threshold are painted in black. Now, the binary image contains the pupil and a few other dark spots from lashes and eyebrows.

The next step is to find the largest connected component i.e., the pupil in this image. One way is to process the entire image to detect the largest connected component. This method is suitable when the head pose is not fixed. However, if the head pose is stable, a small region can be chosen within which the pupil can be located and process that region only in every frame. This reduces a significant amount of computational effort and time required to detect the pupil. To find the largest connected component, the scan plus array based union find (SAUF) algorithm (Lifeng & Yuyanchao 2009) is used. Once the pupil is detected, the centroid of the pupil will give the (x, y) coordinate of the center of the pupil. The bright pupil effect follows the same principle except for the fact that the pupil appears bright and hence the threshold effect is to be applied in such a way that only the bright regions remain. The rest of the procedure is the same as that of the dark pupil effect. The proposed method is depicted in the flowchart in Figure 11.4.

11.2.2 Obtaining a Point of Gaze from a Pupil Coordinate

The pupil coordinate will provide the information on the location of the pupil in any captured frame. However, the goal of detecting the pupil coordinate is to calculate a point of gaze from it. For this purpose, a personal calibration routine is run for every session. A calibration routine typically displays a few points or dots in a particular order or in a random manner. The users are instructed to fixate on those points and while doing so, the corresponding pupil coordinate for each point is recorded. This data is used to obtain a modeling function that gives the relation between pupil coordinates and actual screen coordinates. If (S_x, S_y) are the screen coordinates and (e_x, e_y) are the pupil center coordinates, then two separate functions can be used to relate screen coordinates to pupil coordinates (Equations 11.1 and 11.2):

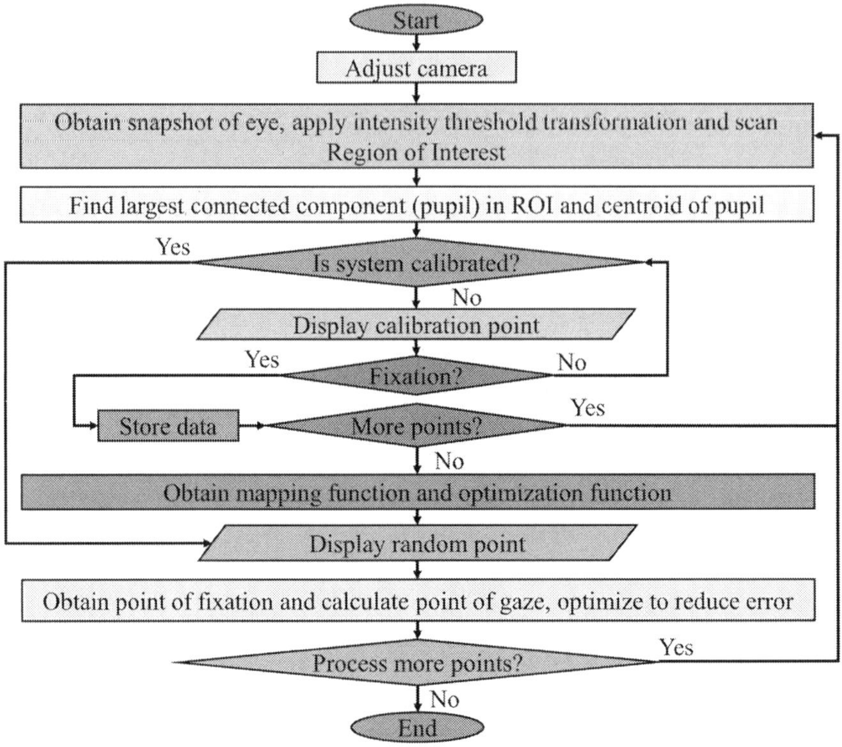

FIGURE 11.4 The proposed method for pupil detection.

$$S_x = f_x(e_x, e_y) \tag{11.1}$$

$$S_y = f_y(e_x, e_y) \tag{11.2}$$

The functions f_x and f_y are modeled as polynomials in e_x, e_y and are represented in Equations 11.3 and 11.4 (Panigrahi & Tripathy 2002):

$$S_x = a_0 + a_1 e_x + a_2 e_y + a_3 e_x e_y \tag{11.3}$$

$$S_y = b_0 + b_1 e_x + b_2 e_y + b_3 e_x e_y \tag{11.4}$$

To compute the actual coordinates (S_x, S_y) for corresponding pupil coordinates (e_x, e_y), we have computed the value of the polynomial coefficients ($a_0, \ldots a_3$) and ($b_0, \ldots b_3$) using regression techniques. The two most popular regression techniques are polynomial affine transformation (Panigrahi & Tripathy 2002) using matrix inversion and the least squares technique. In polynomial affine transformation, four equations are obtained by substituting the recorded data by displaying four different points on the screen and the corresponding pupil coordinates. These equations are solved using the matrix inversion method to obtain unknowns i.e., $(a_0, \ldots a_3)$ and $(b_0, \ldots b_3)$. The other method is to display any number of screen coordinates and pupil coordinates and obtain the values of coefficients (a_0, a_3) and (b_0, b_3) using the least squares method. The values of computed coefficients are used to estimate a new point of gaze on the screen (S_x, S_y), corresponding to any pupil coordinate (e_x, e_y). A detailed implementation and mathematical rigor of PAT (polynomial affine transformation) for registration of satellite images with a map by removing geometric errors is discussed by Panigrahi and Tripathy (2002).

11.3 CALIBRATION SEQUENCE

The experimental setup consists of a screen displaying the scene in which a fixation graph is to be identified. A customized web camera was mounted on a chin rest to obtain snapshots of the eyes. The camera was modified to detect infrared light by removing the IR blocking filter from its lens assembly. The chin rest acts as a support to stabilize head movement of the subject.

As depicted in Figure 11.5, the screen is placed at a distance of 50 cm from the subject's eye. The overall display resolution for the scene is 800 × 600 pixels. The scene is 22 cm in height and 35 cm wide. This provides a visual cone with 25° vertical and 39° horizontal field of view and hence the resolution of the visual angle is 26 pixels per degree vertically and 21 pixels per degree horizontally. IR LEDs were used to illuminate the eyes of the subject.

The first step in calibration was to match the coordinate system of the eye with the coordinate system of the screen. In order to achieve this, a crosshair is displayed on the screen. The subject is instructed to fixate on the center of the crosshair and the camera is adjusted such that the center of the pupil is exactly at

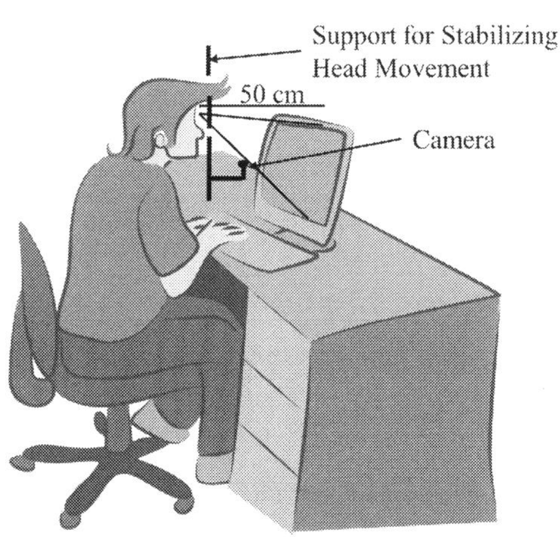

FIGURE 11.5 Experimental setup for gaze estimation.

the center of the crosshair displayed on the screen. Then, calibration is done by repeating the fixate process using a set of 17 random points on the screen in two phases. During the first phase, these points are displayed on the screen as light grey dots. The subject is instructed to fixate on these points and whenever a fixation is detected, the corresponding pupil position is recorded. The light grey dots in Figure 11.6 represent actual screen coordinates and the dark grey dots represent their corresponding pupil coordinates.

These coordinate pairs recorded in the first phase are used to establish the PAT by computing the coefficients of the polynomial. These polynomial coefficients are used to estimate a point of gaze on the screen using Equations 11.3 and 11.4. The second phase is added to improve the accuracy of this estimation. During this phase, the estimated points of gaze and the actual screen coordinates computed using the PAT are used in polynomial regression to obtain a function to optimize the estimated point of gaze. The light grey dots in Figure 11.6 represent the actual screen coordinates and the dark grey dots represent the estimated points of gaze.

11.4 CASE STUDY AND ANALYSIS

The screen was placed 50 cm away from the subject's eye. The overall display resolution for displaying the scene was 800 × 600 pixels. The scene was 22 cm high and 35 cm wide. The angles subtended by the eye vertically and horizontally with the scene were measured (Figure 11.7). The vertical angle was 25° and the horizontal angle was 39°. This provides a visual cone with a resolution of 24 pixels per degree vertically and 21 pixels per degree horizontally.

To test the system, five random points were displayed and their corresponding points of gaze were calculated. The average error for each session was calculated using Equation 11.5:

$$E = \sum \sqrt{(xs - xc)^2 + (ys - yc)^2} \tag{11.5}$$

where xs and ys are actual screen coordinates displayed on the screen and xc and yc are calculated points of gaze by the software. The experiment was performed using a matrix inversion technique and least squares method to deduce the mapping function (Panigrahi & Tripathy 2002). The average error in both cases is presented in Table 11.1. The average error was found to be 48 pixels. This corresponds to a 2.105° of visual angle. A sample of the experimental data can be seen in Figure 11.8.

11.5 COMPARISON OF GAZE ESTIMATION METHOD

The performance of the proposed method is compared with state-of-the-art methods presented in Table 11.2. In this section, various methods proposed for the estimation of eye gaze are described and compared. Meyer et al. (2006) used

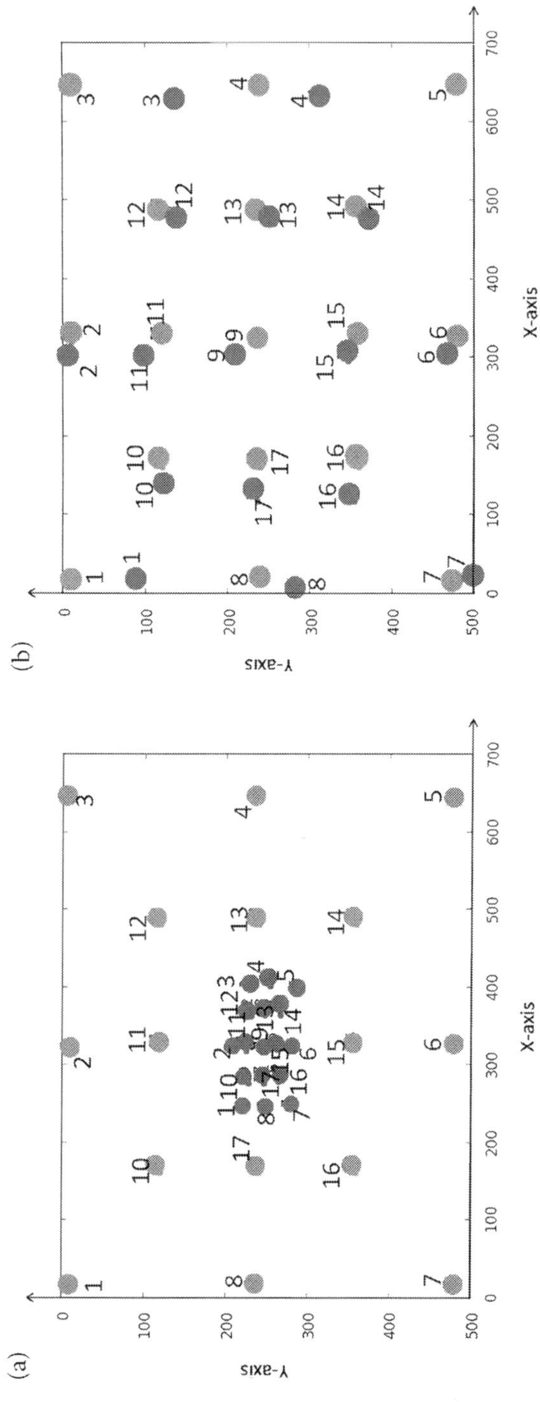

FIGURE 11.6 (a) Phase 1 in calibration; (b) Phase 2 in calibration.

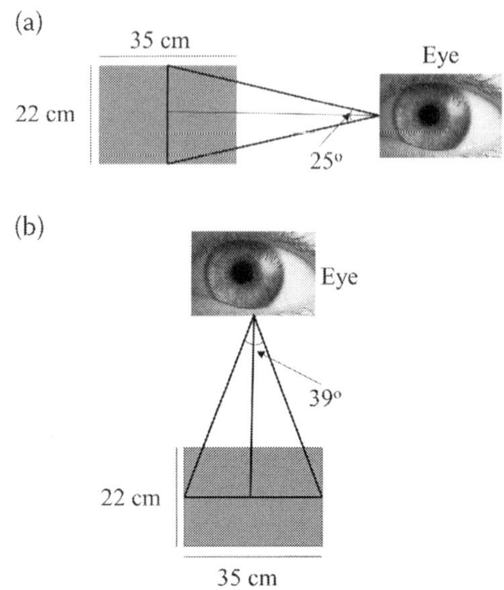

FIGURE 11.7 (a) Vertical visual cone; (b) Horizontal visual cone.

TABLE 11.1
Error analysis of the pupil localization

	Matrix Inversion	**Least Squares**
Horizontal Error	2.8° (59 pixels)	1.81° (38 pixels)
Vertical Error	3.2° (77 pixels)	2.4° (58 pixels)
Mean Error	3.0° (68 pixels)	2.10° (48 pixels)

a high-resolution camera with two infrared light sources and the gaze angle was measured from the offset between corneal reflection and the center of the pupil using bilinear or biquadratic interpolation. The system was tested on simulated data. The method proposed by Hennessey (Hennessey et al 2006) uses a single camera and multiple IR illumination sources.

Shih (Lai et al 2015) uses a hybrid approach in which a glint feature-based model and contour feature-based models are integrated to leverage strengths of both models. Ohno (Ohno & Mukawa 2004) describes a tracking system that allows free head movement by using two cameras for detection of the position of the head in 3D and an IR camera mounted on a pan and tilt mechanism to follow movements of the head. Beymer (Beymer & Flickner 2003) uses four cameras in which two cameras identify head pose and steer the other two cameras for tracking eyes. Zhu (Zhu & Ji 2007) uses two cameras to track eye gaze and

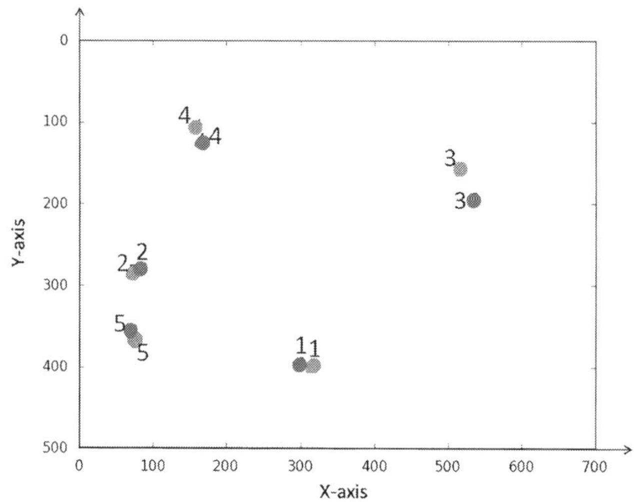

FIGURE 11.8 Test case for gaze estimation.

dynamically compensate for free head movement. Blignaut (2013) uses a system of a single camera with one IR illumination source and evaluates the system for various degrees of polynomial function for regression. Cherif (Cherif et al 2002) introduces a new way in which photo transistors are used instead of a camera. Ji (Lai et al 2015) uses a generalized regression neural network for calibration. Chuang (Jian-nan et al 2009) uses a nonlinear polynomial regression for gaze estimation and generalized regression neural networks for head movement compensation. Table 11.2 represents the overview of comparisons of various eye tracking algorithms and the method proposed.

11.6 SUMMARY

The presented system uses only one feature of the eye i.e., the center of the pupil of the eye of the subject to obtain the point of gaze on a digital screen. This reduces computational effort required for detecting other features such as eye corners, corneal reflections, and glints, enabling high-speed gaze tracking. Also, noise in detection of these additional features is eliminated, thereby increasing the confidence and reliability of the data acquired from our system. As the proposed system uses a simple web camera, the cost of the system is lower than many other eye trackers while achieving accuracies similar to that of expensive methods. The future directions of this research can be multi-front (Kar & Corcoran 2017). Specifically, the future research includes integration of the proposed system in a smart healthcare framework (Sundaravadivel et al 2018).

TABLE 11.2
Comparison of various eye tracking algorithms

Method Used and Reference Literature	Hardware Setup	Features Required	Accuracy
3D Geometrical model (Meyer et al 2006)	Two IR LEDs and one camera	Glints and pupil center	About 1° (on simulated data)
3D Geometrical model (Hennessey et al 2006)	Multiple IR illumination sources, one camera	Pupil contour using bright pupil effect and glints using dark pupil effect	0.90°
3D Geometrical model (Lai et al 2015)	Two cameras and four IR LEDs	Pupil contour and glints	1.18°–1.43°
3D Geometrical model (Ohno & Mukawa 2004)	Two cameras for face detection and one camera on pan and tilt mechanism	3D facial orientation, glints, and pupil contour	About 1°
3D Geometrical model (Beymer & Flickner 2003)	One camera for face detection and two cameras with mirrors on pan and tilt mechanism	3D facial orientation, glints, and pupil contour	0.6°
3D Geometrical model (Zhu & Ji 2007)	Two cameras with multiple IR illumination sources	Pupil and glints	1.6°
2D Regression (Blignaut 2013)	One camera, one IR LED	Pupil and glints	1.17°
2D Regression (Cherif et al 2002)	Photo transistors, pulsed IR illumination	No image is used	2.5°
2D Regression (Jian-nan et al 2009)	Two concentric rings of IR LEDs, one camera	Pupil and glints	5°–8°
2D Regression (Hansen & Dan 2010)	Two loops of IR LEDs and one camera	Pupil and glints	20 pixels
2D Regression, the proposed method	Modified web camera with built in IR LEDs and IR blocking filter removed	Pupil center only	2.10°

Exercises

1. What are the applications of point gaze estimation?
2. What are EOG and VOG and EEG? Give differences between EOG and EEG.

3. What is active imaging and passive imaging in the context of pupil imaging?
4. What is a dark pupil and bright pupil effect in occulography?
5. Draw a flowchart elucidating the flow of extracting the pupil from an image.
6. What is PAT (polynomial affine transformation)?
7. How do you calibrate and plot the point of gaze fixation with that of the screen coordinate?
8. Give a brief comparison of the prevailing state of gaze estimation method or algorithm.

REFERENCES

Beymer, D & Flickner, M 2003, 'Eye gaze tracking using an active stereo head,' in *Proceedings of the 2003 IEEE Computer Society Conference on Computer Vision and Pattern Recognition*, vol. 2, no. 2, p. II-451–8.

Blignaut, P 2013, 'Mapping the pupil-glint vector to gaze coordinates in a simple video-based eye tracker,' *Journal of Eye Movement Research*, vol. 7, no. 1, pp. 1–11.

Bulling, A 2011 April, 'Eye movement analysis for activity recognition using electro-oculography,' IEEE Transactions on Pattern Analysis and Machine Intelligence, vol. 33, no. 4, pp. 741–753.

Cherif, ZR, Nait-Ali, A, Motsch, JF & Krebs, MO 2002, 'An adaptive calibration of an infrared light device used for gaze tracking,' in *Proceedings of the 19th IEEE Instrumentation and Measurement Technology Conference*, vols. 1, 2, no. May, pp. 1029–1033.

Corcoran, PM et al. 2012 May, 'Real-time eye gaze tracking for gaming design and consumer electronics systems,' *IEEE Transactions on Consumer Electronics*, vol. 58, no. 2, pp. 347–355.

Crane, HD & Steele, CM 1985, 'Generation-V dual-Purkinje-image eyetracker,' *Applied Optics*, vol. 24, no. 4, pp. 527–537.

Duchowski, AT 2002, 'A breath-first survey of eye-tracking applications,' *Behavior Research Methods, Instruments, & Computers*, vol. 34, no. 4, pp. 455–470.

Guestrin, ED & Eizenman, M 2006 June, 'General theory of remote gaze estimation using the pupil center and corneal reflections', *IEEE Transactions on Biomedical Engineering*, vol. 53, no. 6, pp. 1124–1133.

Hansen, W & Dan, QJ 2010 March, 'In the eye of the beholder: A survey of models for eyes and gaze,' *IEEE Transactions on Pattern Analysis and Machine Intelligence*, vol. 32, no. 3, pp. 478–500.

Hennessey, C, Noureddin, B & Lawrence, P 2006, 'A single camera eye-gaze tracking system with free head motion,' *Measurement*, vol. 1, no. March, pp. 27–29.

Jian-Nan, C, Chuang, Z, Yan-Tao, Y, Yang, L & Han, Z 2009, 'Eye gaze calculation based on nonlinear polynomial and generalized regression neural network,' in *Proceedings of the 5th International Conference on National Computing, 14–16 Aug. 2009, Tianjian, China*, pp. 617–623.

Kar, A & Corcoran, P 2017, 'A review and analysis of eye-gaze estimation systems, algorithms and performance evaluation methods in consumer platforms,' *IEEE Access*, vol. 5, pp. 16495–16519.

Lai, CC, Shih, SW & Hung, YP 2015, 'Hybrid method for 3-D gaze tracking using glint and contour features,' *IEEE Transactions on Circuits and Systems for Video Technology*, vol. 25, no. 1, pp. 24–37.

Lee, HC, Luong, DT, Cho, CW, Lee, EC & Park, KR 2010 November, 'Gaze tracking system at a distance for controlling IPTV,' *IEEE Transactions on Consumer Electronics*, vol. 56, no.4, pp. 2577–2583.

Levine, JL 1981, *An Eye-Controlled Computer*, Research Report RC-8857, IBM Thomas J. Watson Research Center, Yorktown Heights, NY.

Lifeng, H & Yuyanchao, KS 2009 September, 'Fast connected-component labelling,' *Pattern Recognition*, vol. 42, no. 9, pp. 1977–1987.

Meyer, A, Böhme, M, Martinetz, T & Barth, E 2006, 'A single-camera remote eye tracker,' *Perception and Interactive Technologies*, vol. 4021, pp. 208–211.

Ohno, T & Mukawa, N 2004, 'A free-head, simple calibration, gaze tracking system that enables gaze-based interaction,' in *Proceedings of the 2004 Symposium on Eye Tracking Research & Applications – ETRA'2004, 22–24, 2004, San Antonio, Texas, USA*, pp. 115–122.

Panigrahi, N & Tripathy, S 2002 July, 'Image registration using polynomial affine transformation,' *Defence Science Journal*, vol. 52, no. 3, pp. 5253–5259.

Robinson, DA 1963 October, 'A method of measuring eye movement using a scleral search coil in a magnetic field,' *IEEE Transactions on Bio-Medical Electronics*, vol. 10, no. 4, pp. 137–145.

Sugioka, A, Ebisawa, Y & Ohtani, M 1996, 'Noncontant video-based eye-gaze detection method allowing large head displacements,' in *Proceedings of the International Conference on Medicine and Biology Society, 31 Oct.–3 Nov. 1996, Amsterdam, Netherlands,*, pp. 526–528.

Sundaravadivel, P, Kougianos, E, Mohanty, SP & Ganapathiraju, M 2018 January, 'Everything you wanted to know about smart healthcare,' *IEEE Consumer Electronics Magazine (CEM)*, vol. 8, no. 1, pp. 18–28.

Wang, JG & Sung, E 2002 June, 'Study on eye gaze estimation,' *IEEE Transactions on Systems, Man, and Cybernetics – Part B*, vol. 32, no. 3, pp. 332–350.

Yoo, DH & Chung, MJ 2005 April, 'A novel non-intrusive eye gaze estimation using cross-ratio under large head motion,' *Computer Vision and Image Understanding*, vol. 98, no. 1, pp. 25–51.

Zhu, Z & Ji, Q 2007, 'Novel eye gaze tracking techniques under natural head movement,' *IEEE Transactions on Biomedical Engineering*, vol. 54, no. 12, pp. 2246–2260.

Zhu, J & Yang, J 2012, 'Evaluation of pupil center-eye corner vector for gaze estimation using a web cam,' in *Proceedings of the Symposium on Eye Tracking Research and Applications*, pp. 217–220.

12 Detection of Epileptic Seizures from EEG Data

OVERVIEW

Epilepsy is a neurological disorder emanating from within the central nervous system or parietal zone of the human brain. In epilepsy, the activity of the brain becomes abnormal, causing seizures or periods of unusual behavior, sensations, and sometimes loss of awareness. Therefore, detection of epileptic seizures is very important for a proper diagnosis of epilepsy. Some of the causes of epilepsy are (a) low oxygen during birth, (b) head injuries that occur during birth or due to injury to the brain, (c) brain tumors, (d) genetic conditions that result in brain injury, and (e) infections such as meningitis or encephalitis, etc.

Some generic symptoms and signs of epilepsy seizures are (a) temporary confusion, (b) a staring spell, (c) uncontrollable jerking movements of the arms and legs, (d) loss of consciousness or awareness, (e) cognitive or emotional symptoms, such as fear, anxiety, or feelings of deja vu, etc.

A sizable population are epileptic patients and undergo the trauma of unpredictable seizures. The study of an EEG of a patient by a trained doctor to diagnose the abnormal pattern from the EEG forms the basis of diagnosis of epilepsy. This chapter discusses the current state of the art in identification and diagnosis of epilepsy, features generally found in the EEG signal, or the derived properties that together form a feature vector to classify and identify epilepsy from a normal EEG. Methods and tools are required to make an epilepsy classification and identification system.

12.1 INTRODUCTION

Epilepsy is a common brain disorder that, according to an estimate of the World Health Organization, affects almost 60 million people around the world. Epilepsy is characterized by the recurrent and sudden incidence of epileptic seizures that can lead to dangerous and possibly life-threatening situations (Iasemidis 2003; Buck et al 1997). The seizures are the result of a transient and unexpected electrical disturbance of the brain and excessive neuronal discharge that is evident in the electroencephalogram (EEG) signal. Consequently, the EEG signal has been the most utilized signal in clinical assessments of the state of the brain and detection of epileptic seizures, and is very important for a proper diagnosis of epilepsy. The detection of epileptic seizures by visual scanning of a patient's EEG data usually collected over a few days is a tedious and

DOI: 10.1201/9781003241386-12

time-consuming process. In addition, it requires a domain expert to analyze the entire length of the EEG recordings in order to detect epileptic activity.

Therefore, devising a reliable automatic classification and EEG detection system is of significant importance, which would ensure a reliable diagnosis of epilepsy. It will significantly improve the diagnosis of epilepsy as well as long-term monitoring and treatment of patients. For example, long-term treatment with anti-epileptic drugs, which may cause cognitive or other neurological side effects, could be reduced to a targeted short-acting intervention (Elger 2001). Therefore, there is a strong demand for the development of such automated systems, due to increased use of long-term EEG recordings for proper valuation and treatment of neurological diseases, including epilepsy. Also, it will significantly reduce the cost of diagnosis, lessening the financial burden to the patient. The possibility of the expert misreading the data and failing to make a proper decision would also be narrowed down (Guler & Ubeyli 2005; Webber et al 1993).

12.2 PRESENT STATE OF THE ART

The detection of epileptic seizures by visual scanning of a patient's EEG data usually collected over a few days is a tedious and time-consuming process. In addition, it requires an expert to analyze the entire length of the EEG recordings, in order to detect epileptic activity. A reliable automatic classification and detection system would ensure a timely treatment. Often long-term monitoring and diagnosis of epilepsy as well as its treatment significantly improves the condition of the patients. For example, the long-term treatment with anti-epileptic drugs, which may cause cognitive or other neurological side effects, could be reduced to a targeted short-acting intervention (Elger 2001). Therefore, there is a strong demand for the development of automated systems to diagnose, classify, and detect elliptic seizures. The automatic scanning, classification, and detection of epileptic seizures will help in proper evaluation and treatment of epilepsy, including other neurological diseases. It will eliminate and minimize the possibility of the expert misreading the data and failing to make a proper decision; also, it can reduce the financial burden of treatment.

Automatic classification and detection of seizures from EEG data has been studied by many researchers using many different approaches. Significant among such developments are by Gotman (Gotman 1982), who presented a computerized system for detecting a variety of seizures, while Qu and Gotman (Qu & Gotman 1997) proposed the use of the nearest-neighbor classifier on EEG features extracted in both time and frequency domains to detect the onset of epileptic seizures. Artificial neural network–based detection systems for diagnosis of epilepsy have been proposed by several researchers (Ubeyli 2006; Tzallas et al 2007).

The method uses the feature vector containing values, average EEG amplitude, average EEG duration, variation coefficient, dominant frequency, and average power spectrum, as inputs to an adaptive neural network. The method uses a raw EEG signal as an input to extract the learning vector through quantization and processing of the EEG signal acquired from the subject. In a new neural network model called LAMSTAR (large memory storage and retrieval), the network and two time-domain attributes of EEG; namely, relative spike amplitude and spike rhythmicity as inputs for the purpose of detecting seizures. The algorithm proposed by Kiymik et al. [18] uses a backpropagation neural network with periodogram and autoregressive (AR) features as input for automatic detection of epileptic seizures. A classification methodology based on wavelet analysis and both radial basis function and Levenberg-Marquardt backpropagation neural network is used for learning and classification. Wavelet analysis and mixture of experts, in addition to the artificial neural network, are used to classify EEG signals and detect seizures. The methods clearly establish the fact that the approaches used in classification and identification of epilepsy from EEG data follow a pattern of analysis that is depicted in the block diagram (Figure 12.1).

12.3 CLASSIFICATION OF EEG DATA

From the perspective of epilepsy in particular and abnormality in general, the EEG data can be classified into three subject groups: a) healthy subjects (normal EEG), b) epileptic subjects during a seizure-free interval (interictal EEG), and c) epileptic subjects during a seizure (ictal EEG). The EEG signal classification and seizure detection problem is modeled as a three-group classification problem that is of great clinical significance. An automated system able to accurately differentiate between normal and interictal EEG signals can be used to diagnose epilepsy, while a system that can accurately differentiate between interictal and ictal EEG signals can be used to detect seizures in a clinical setting. Therefore, the classification algorithm must be able to classify all three groups accurately and at the same time be robust with respect to EEG signal variations across various mental states and subjects. The improvement of the classification accuracy is mainly based on the design of both an appropriate feature space, by identifying combinations of all extracted features that increase the inter-class separation, and classifiers that can accurately classify all three groups of EEG signals based on the selected and reduced feature space. Real EEG recordings were applied to test algorithm performance and the results indicated that the algorithm has a special potential to be applied within an automatic epilepsy diagnosis system.

The hierarchical tree depicting classification of EEG signals into various classes and subclasses is depicted (Figure 12.2). An EEG classifier capable of classifying all of these classes and subclasses needs to be trained for different feature sets. The feature sets need to be obtained from the EEG database automatically and sanitized or reduced in such a manner that they portray a high intra-class variance and low inter-class/subclass variance. A possible set of features for the best classification is average frequency, average EEG amplitude, average EEG duration, variation coefficient, dominant frequency, and average power spectrum.

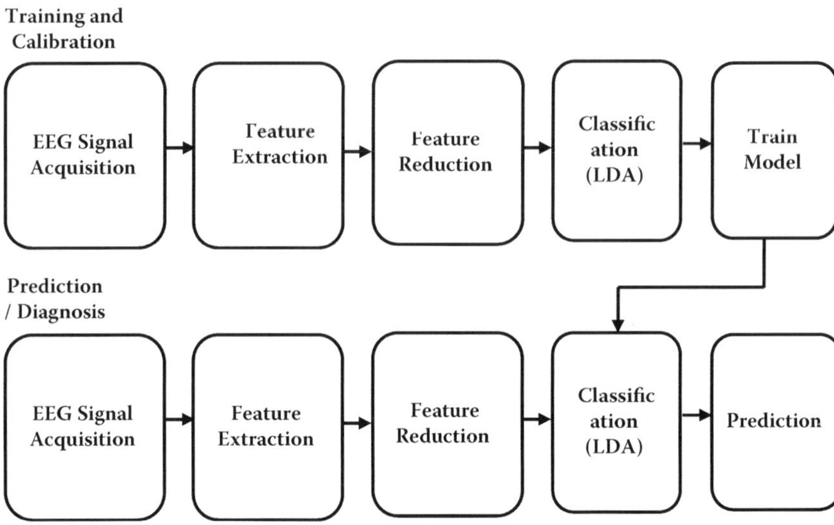

FIGURE 12.1 Pattern of EEG data analysis using signal classification and machine learning.

12.4 DESIGNING AN AUTOMATIC EPILEPTIC SEIZURE DETECTION SYSTEM

In this section, we discuss the design of an automatic seizure detection system. The material and the methods required to realize such a system has many options to choose from. The tools require classifying and isolating the EEG data corresponding to the seizure.

12.4.1 Materials

To design a classifier, the first ingredient that is necessary is a large amount of tagged data. The EEG data used for designing our system constitutes EEG data corresponding to both normal and epileptic subjects, made available by Axxonate Networks, Bangalore. A mix of three types of EEG data sets from three different types, healthy subjects with normal EEG data, epileptic subjects during a seizure-free interval with interictal EEG data, and epileptic subjects during a seizure with ictal (epileptic) EEG data, are considered. Each data set is recorded with a 64-channel EEG acquisition system with a 25 s duration. These segments were selected and cut out from the continuous multi-channel EEG recordings after visual inspection for artifacts (e.g., saccade, fix, and blink due to muscle activity or eye movement). The first EEG data set corresponds to healthy subjects, who were relaxed in an awakened state, using the standardized electrode placement technique. The second and third data sets were obtained from five different epileptic subjects during a seizure-free and seizure interval,

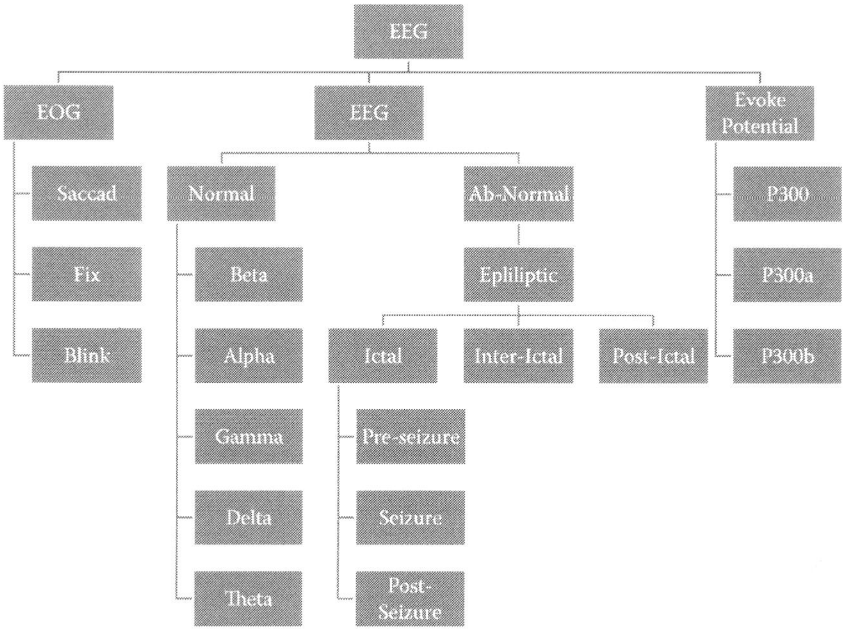

FIGURE 12.2 A generic classification of an EEG signal.

respectively, were taken from the intracranial EEG recordings during pre-surgical diagnosis.

Epilepsy is considered as a phenomena emanating from the temporal lobe of the brain and is diagnosed as temporal lobe epilepsy as the epileptogenic focus being hippocampal formation. A schematic of an intracranial electrode placement is shown in Figure 12.3(b). The depth electrode was implanted symmetrically into the hippocampal formations and the strip electrodes were implanted onto the lateral and basal regions of the neocortex (Figure 12.3(b)). The EEG segments selected from all the recording sites exhibit ictal activity. Each EEG segment is considered as a separate EEG signal, resulting in a sizable number of EEG data segments.

There are five broad spectral sub-bands of the EEG signal that are generally of clinical interest: delta (0–4 Hz), theta (4–8 Hz), alpha (8–16 Hz), beta (16–32 Hz), and gamma waves (32–64 Hz). Higher frequencies are often more common in abnormal brain states such as epilepsy (i.e., there is a shift of EEG signal energy from lower- to higher-frequency bands before and during a seizure). These five frequency sub-bands provide more accurate information about neuronal activities underlying the problem and, consequently, some changes in the EEG signal that are not so obvious in the original full-spectrum signal, can be amplified when each sub-band is considered independently. That is the basic premise of seizure classification of an EEG signal. Most of the features were extracted from each sub-band separately, after wavelet decomposition of the

(a)

(b)

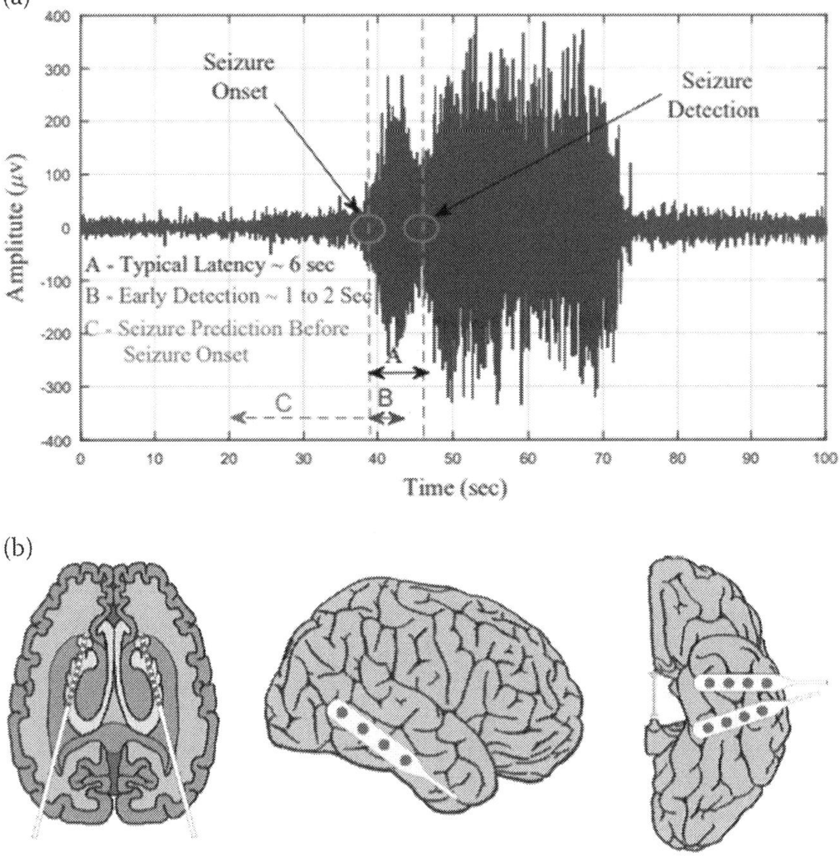

FIGURE 12.3 (a) Time domain analysis of an epileptic seizure; (b) Implanted intracranial electrodes for detection of epilepsy.

full-spectrum EEG signal, as well as reconstructed in all five sub-bands using the inverse wavelet transform.

For example, the difference between normal and interictal EEG data is more apparent in Figure 12.3(b), where only theta sub-bands are presented, than in Figure 12.2, where the same but full-spectrum signals are shown. On the other hand, ictal EEG data are easier to distinguish, mainly due to higher amplitudes.

As an example, the first 5 s of all three different EEG data segments are magnified and shown in Figure 12.3(a). Interictal EEG data can contain only occasional transient waveforms, as isolated spikes, spike trains, sharp waves, or spike-wave complexes, while ictal EEG date are composed of a continuous discharge of polymorphic waveforms of variable amplitude and frequency, spike and sharp wave complexes, rhythmic hypersynchrony, or electrocerebral inactivity observed over a duration longer than the average duration of these abnormalities during interictal periods, as shown in Figure 12.3(a).

12.4.2 Methods

In this section, an automated classification of EEG signals for the detection of epileptic seizures based on wavelet transform and statistical pattern recognition is discussed. The method is depicted in in the flowchart in Figure 12.4.

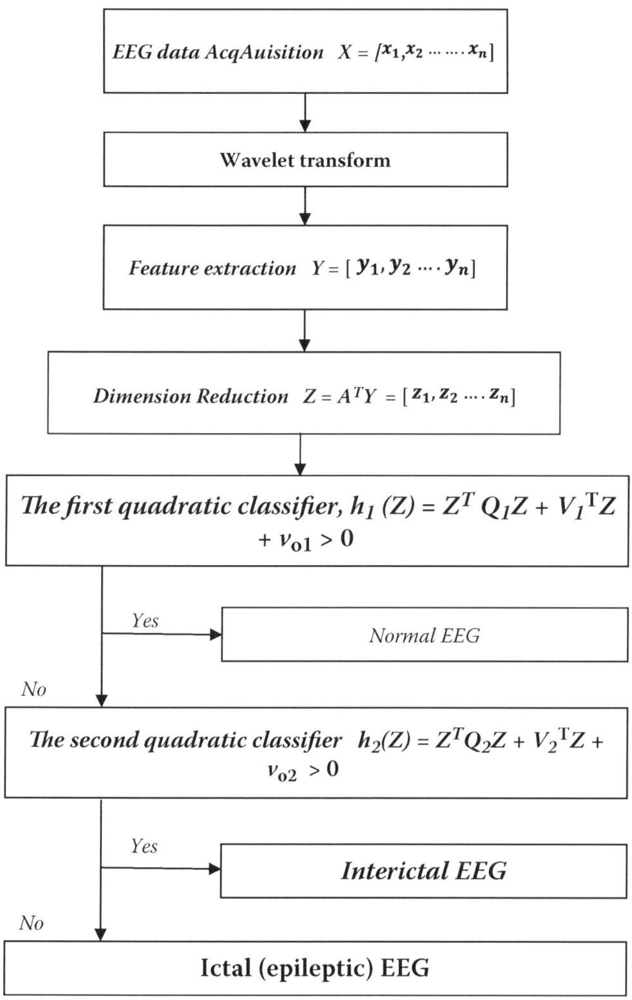

FIGURE 12.4 Process flow of classification algorithm.

Step 1. The first step of this method is to obtain a set of features after wavelet transform of EEG data, including energy, entropy, and standard deviation of both wavelet coefficients and the EEG signal in different frequency bands of clinical interest.

Step 2. The second step is to perform dimension reduction of the feature space using scatter matrices.

Step 3. Finally, two quadratic classifiers are designed that are able to distinguish all three groups of EEG signals of interest from each other. The entire flow of the algorithm is shown in Figure 12.4.

12.4.3 Wavelet Transform

Abnormalities in EEG data during serious neurological diseases such as epilepsy are too subtle to be detected using conventional techniques that usually transform mostly qualitative diagnostic criteria into a more objective quantitative signal feature classification problem. The techniques that have been applied to address this problem include the analysis of EEG signals for the detection of epileptic seizures using the autocorrelation function, time domain features, frequency domain features, time-frequency analysis, nonlinear time series analysis, and wavelet transform. However, the results of various studies have demonstrated that the wavelet transform is the most promising method for extracting features from EEG signals (Guler & Ubeyli 2005; Adeli et al 2004). As such, the wavelet transform is used to extract features from EEG signals.

The wavelet transform, as a liner time-frequency transform, represents an efficient analytical tool in signal processing, pattern recognition and classification, and is suitable for analysis of transient and non-stationary phenomena as well as noise reduction. As a class of functions, it has the ability to localize information in both time and frequency. Therefore, the wavelet transform has been utilized widely in biomedical signal processing. Using discrete wavelet analysis, a multi-resolution description is used to decompose a given signal x(t) into increasingly finer detail based on two sets of basis functions, the wavelets and the scaling functions, given by Equation 12.1:

$$x(t) = \sum_k 2^{j_0/2} a_{j0}(k)\varphi(2^{j0}t - k) + \sum_{j-j_0}^{\infty} \sum_k 2^{j/2} d_j(k)\, \psi\, (2^j t - k) \quad (12.1)$$

where functions $\varphi(t)$ and $\psi(t)$ are the basic scaling and mother wavelet, respectively. In the expansion, the first summation represents an approximation of $x(t)$ based on the scale index of j_0, while the second term adds more detail using larger j (finer scales). The coefficients in this wavelet expansion are called the discrete wavelet transform (DWT) of the signal (t). When the wavelets are orthogonal, these coefficients can be calculated by (Equation 12.2):

$$d_j(k) = \int_{-\infty}^{\infty} 2^{j/2} x(t)\, \psi\, (2^j t - k) dt \quad (12.2)$$

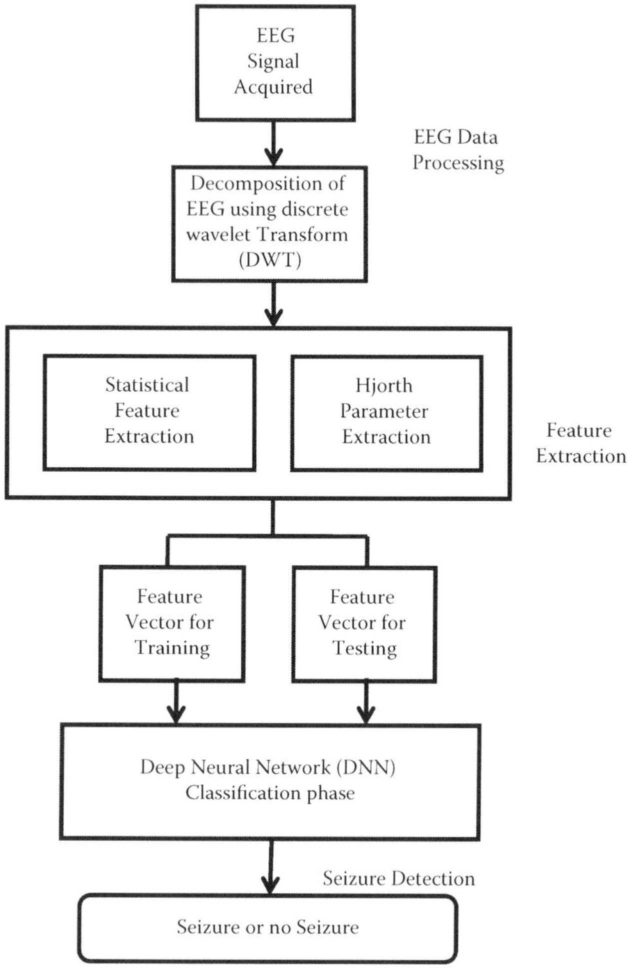

FIGURE 12.5 Flow chart of the Seizure detection process.

where $a_j(k)$ and $d_j(k)$ are the wavelet approximation and detail coefficients, respectively.

In the DWT, the frequency axis is divided into dyadic intervals towards the lower frequencies, while the bandwidth length decreases exponentially. The wavelet packet (WP) transform is a generalization of the DWT in which decomposition is undertaken in both directions (lower and higher frequencies). This general decomposition offers a greater range of possibilities for signal analysis than the discrete wavelet decomposition. In the WP tree, each node is recognized by the decomposition level (scale) l with respect to the WP tree root and the frequency band f. The ability of the wavelet transform in adaptive time-scale representation and decomposition of a signal into different frequency sub-bands presents an efficient signal analysis method without introducing a calculation burden. Based on wavelet coefficients obtained after the wavelet transform, the signal can be reconstructed in each of the previously derived sub-bands and its time-domain features in different sub-bands can be studied separately.

A generic flowchart for the classification of EEG data is depicted in Figure 12.5. The flowchart has three distinct sub-sections: (1) EEG data processing, (2) extraction of features from processed EEG data, and (3) learning of the classifier and classification of EEG signals for the detection of seizures.

12.5 SUMMARY

This chapter discussed the generic classification of EEG data from the point of view of detection of seizures due to epilepsy. The contents of a feature vector that specify a seizure from that of the normal EEG signal were discussed. The methods and tools that are useful in designing a seizure detector were reviewed. Further, how a wavelet transformation and a neural network are used to train and detect seizures from time-varying EEG signals of the subject were discussed. Also, how the coefficients obtained from a discrete wavelet transform were used as the signature vector after reduction was discussed. This vector is used by quadratic classifiers for the classification of the EEG signal into three important clasess normal, interictal, and ictal.

Exercise

1. What is epilepsy? How it is characterized with respect to the EEG signal?
2. What are the prevailing techniques to detect epilepsy from an EEG signal of a subject?
3. Describe various stages of analysis of an EEG signal leading to the classification of EEG data.
4. Give a block diagram and describe the process of pattern analysis of EEG signal classification.
5. Give a generic classification of an EEG signal based on its frequency, amplitude, average power spectrum, average frequency, average EEG amplitude, and dominant frequency.
6. What are the requirements to design an automatic epileptic seizure detection system?
7. Give a step-by-step algorithm for an automatic EEG signal classification leading to the detection of seizures.

REFERENCES

Adeli, H, Ghosh-Dastidar, S & Dadmehr, N 2004, 'A wavelet-chaos methodology for analysis of EEGs and EEG sub-bands to detect seizure and epilepsy,' *IEEE Transactions on Biomedical Engineering*, vol. 54, no. 2, p. 205.

Buck, D, Baker, GA, Jacoby, A, Smith, DF & Chadwick, DW 1997, 'Patient's experiences of injury as a result of epilepsy,' *Epilepsia*, vol. 38, p. 439.

Elger, CE 2001, 'Future trends in epileptology,' *Current Opinion in Neurology*, vol. 14, p. 185.

Gigola, S, Ortiz, F, Attellis, CE, Silvaand, W & Kochen, S 2004, 'Prediction of epileptic seizures using accumulated energy in a multi-resolution framework,' *Journal of Neuroscience Methods*, vol. 38, p. 107.

Gotman, J 1982, 'Automatic recognition of epileptic seizures in the EEG,' *Electroencephalography and Clinical Neurophysiology*, vol. 54, p. 530.

Guler, I & Ubeyli, ED 2005, 'Adaptive neuro fuzzy inference system for classification of EEG signals using wavelet coefficients,' *Journal of Neuroscience Methods*, vol. 148, p. 113.

Iasemidis, LD 2003, 'Epileptic seizure prediction and control,' *IEEE Transactions on Biomedical Engineering*, vol. 50, p. 549.

Qu, H & Gotman, J 1997, 'A patient-specific algorithm for the detection of seizure onset in long-term EEG monitoring: Possible use as a warning device,' *IEEE Transactions on Biomedical Engineering*, vol. 44, no. 2, p. 115.

Tzallas, AT, Tsipouras, MG & Fotiadis, DI 2007, 'Automatic seizure detection based on time frequency analysis and artificial neural networks,' *Computational Intelligence and Neuroscience*, vol. 80510.

Ubeyli, ED 2006, 'Analysis of EEG signals using Lyapunov exponents,' *Neural Network World*, vol. 16, no. 3, p. 257.

Webber, WR, Litt, B, Lesser, RP, Fisher, RS & Bankman, I 1993, 'Automatic EEG spike detection: What should the computer imitate,' *Electroencephalography and Clinical Neurophysiology*, vol. 87, no. 6, p. 364.

Appendix

A1 METHOD TO LOAD THE EEG DATA INTO THE EEGLAB TOOLBOX

To load the data in .edf format to MATLAB®, we have used the EEGLAB toolbox. The source for the toolbox is provided in Software Requirement section. The steps for loading data are as follows:

Step 1. Change current directory to the EEGLAB folder. Add this path and in the MATLAB terminal type: "EEGLAB."

Step 2. A pop-up window will appear; follow the path:

"File » Import data » Using EEGLAB functions and plugins » From EDF/EDF^{+}/GDF files(Biosig toolbox)."

Now locate the .edf file in file explorer and click open to import.

Figure A1 Demonstrates the above path.

Step 3. After the import is complete, load the data as a .mat file.

for use in MATLAB, type:

"A= ALLEEG.data;"

This stores the data in A (as MATLAB array) and lets the user access each channel by slicing the array. For our case, it was 37-channel data, where each row in an array represents one channel data. Note the data is in single format, so double conversion is required. Figure A2 demonstrates this process.

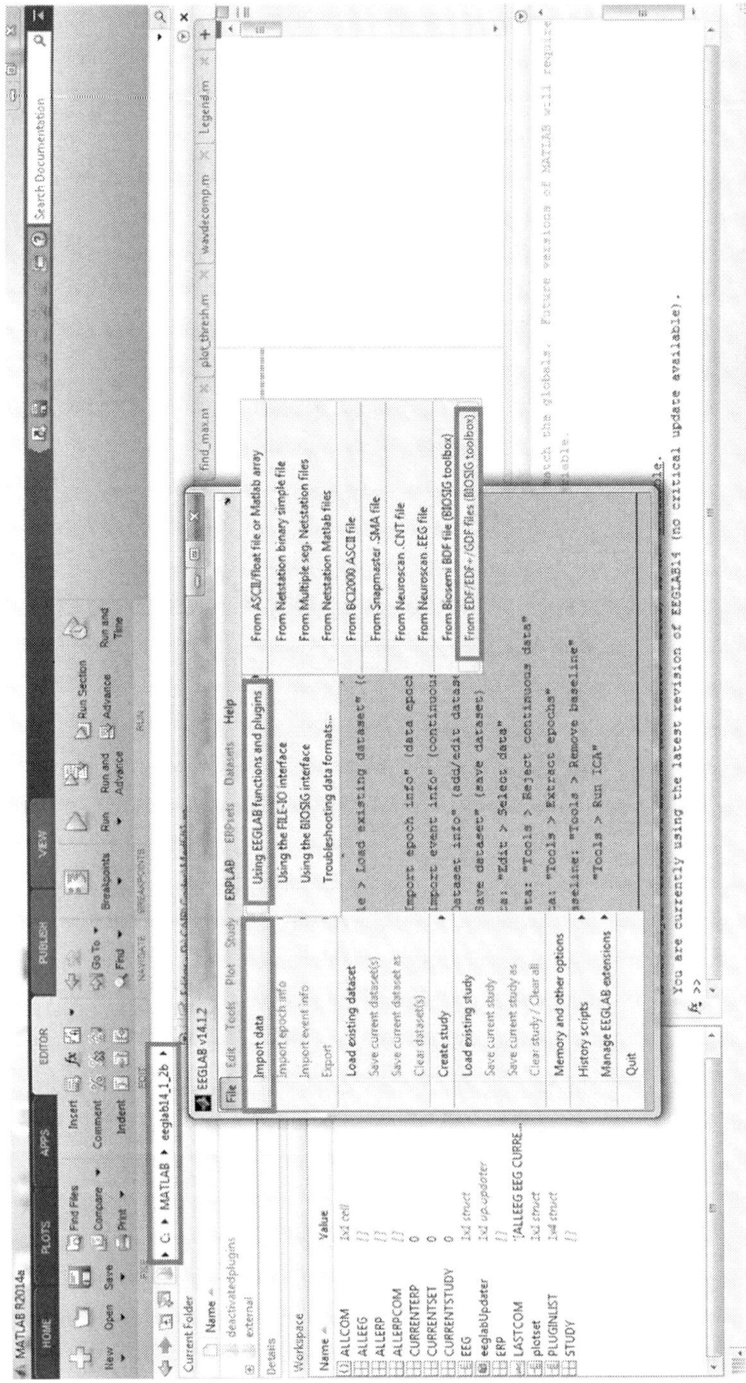

FIGURE A1 Loading .edf data in MATLAB using the EEGLAB toolbox.

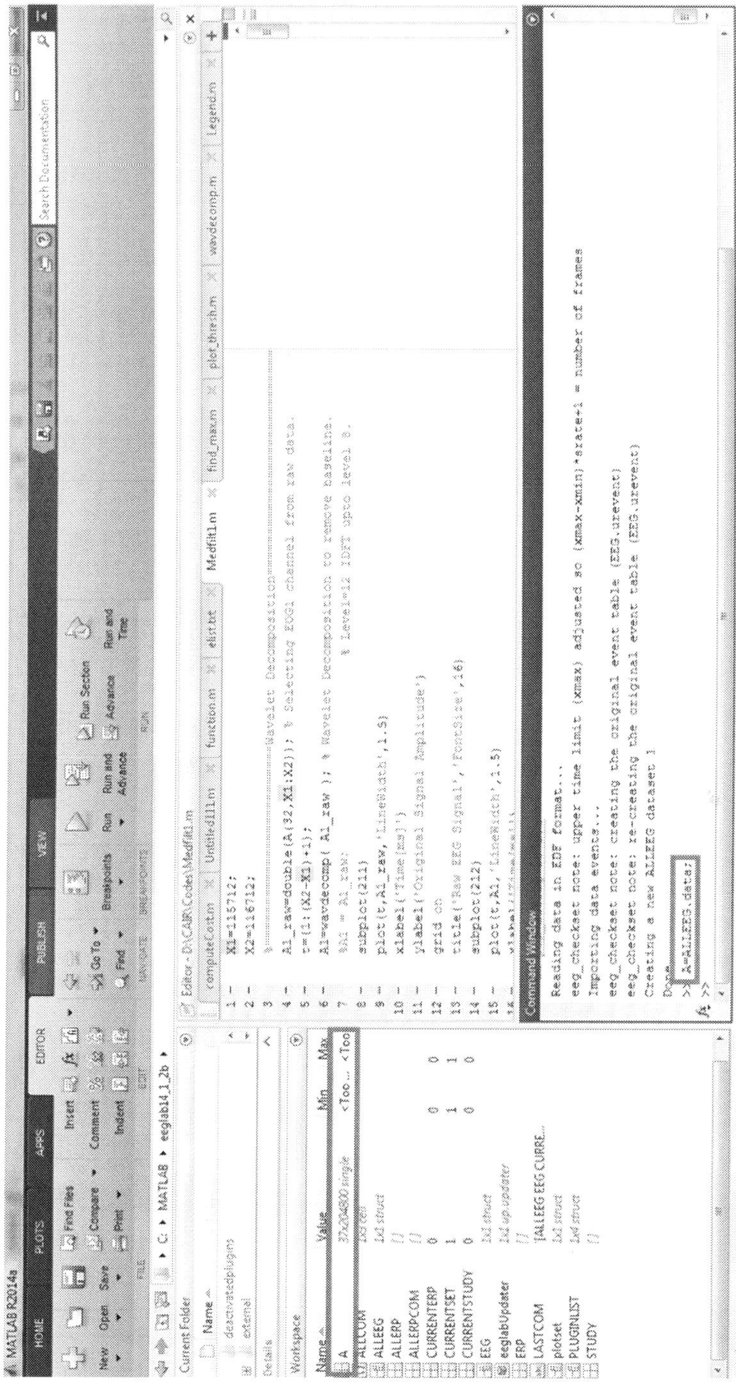

FIGURE A2 Converting the .edf file in MATLAB array.

A2 THIS MATLAB CODE TO PLOTS THE EEG SIGNAL, TO COMPUTE THE WAVELET COEFFICIENT OF GAMMA, BETA, ALPHA, BETA AND DELTA WAVES ARTEFACTS FROM THE EEG SIGNAL. IT PLOTS THE EEG COMPONENTS SEPARATELY. ALSO IT COMPUTES THE OCCURRENCE OF THE MAXIMUM FREQUENCY OF THESE COMPONENTS

```
load eegdata.mat;
s=eegdata;
figure;p=plot(s);
title('EEG Signal')
fs = 500;
% Sampling frequency
N=length(s);
waveletFunction = 'db8';
[C,L] = wavedec(s,8,waveletFunction);
cD1 = detcoef(C,L,1);
cD2 = detcoef(C,L,2);
cD3 = detcoef(C,L,3);
cD4 = detcoef(C,L,4);
cD5 = detcoef(C,L,5); %GAMA
cD6 = detcoef(C,L,6); %BETA
cD7 = detcoef(C,L,7); %ALPHA
cD8 = detcoef(C,L,8); %THETA
cA8 = appcoef(C,L,waveletFunction,8); %DELTA
D1 = wrcoef('d',C,L,waveletFunction,1);
D2 = wrcoef('d',C,L,waveletFunction,2);
D3 = wrcoef('d',C,L,waveletFunction,3);
D4 = wrcoef('d',C,L,waveletFunction,4);
D5 = wrcoef('d',C,L,waveletFunction,5); %GAMMA
D6 = wrcoef('d',C,L,waveletFunction,6); %BETA
D7 = wrcoef('d',C,L,waveletFunction,7); %ALPHA
D8 = wrcoef('d',C,L,waveletFunction,8); %THETA
A8 = wrcoef('a',C,L,waveletFunction,8); %DELTA
Gamma = D5;
figure; subplot(5,1,1); plot(1:1:length(Gamma),Gamma);title('GAMMA');
Beta = D6;
subplot(5,1,2); plot(1:1:length(Beta), Beta); title('BETA');
Alpha = D7;
subplot(5,1,3); plot(1:1:length(Alpha),Alpha); title('ALPHA');
Theta = D8;
subplot(5,1,4); plot(1:1:length(Theta),Theta);title('THETA');
D8 = detrend(D8,0);
Delta = A8;
%figure, plot(0:1/fs:1,Delta);
```

```
subplot(5,1,5);plot(1:1:length(Delta),Delta);title('DELTA');
D5 = detrend(D5,0);
xdft = fft(D5);
freq = 0:N/length(D5):N/2;
xdft = xdft(1:length(D5)/2+1);
figure;subplot(511);plot(freq,abs(xdft));title('GAMMA-FREQUENCY');
[~,I] = max(abs(xdft));
fprintf('Gamma:Maximum occurs at %3.2fHz.\n',freq(I));
D6 = detrend(D6,0);
xdft2 = fft(D6);
freq2 = 0:N/length(D6):N/2;
xdft2 = xdft2(1:length(D6)/2+1);
% figure;
subplot(512);plot(freq2,abs(xdft2));title('BETA');
[~,I] = max(abs(xdft2));
fprintf('Beta:Maximum occurs at %3.2fHz.\n',freq2(I));
D7 = detrend(D7,0);
xdft3 = fft(D7);
freq3 = 0:N/length(D7):N/2;
xdft3 = xdft3(1:length(D7)/2+1);
% figure;
subplot(513);plot(freq3,abs(xdft3));title('ALPHA');
[~,I] = max(abs(xdft3));
fprintf('Alpha:Maximum occurs at %f Hz.\n',freq3(I));
xdft4 = fft(D8);
freq4 = 0:N/length(D8):N/2;
xdft4 = xdft4(1:length(D8)/2+1);
% figure;
subplot(514);plot(freq4,abs(xdft4));title('THETA');
[~,I] = max(abs(xdft4));
fprintf('Theta:Maximum occurs at %f Hz.\n',freq4(I));
A8 = detrend(A8,0);
xdft5 = fft(A8);
freq5 = 0:N/length(A8):N/2;
xdft5 = xdft5(1:length(A8)/2+1);
% figure;
subplot(515);plot(freq3,abs(xdft5));title('DELTA');
[~,I] = max(abs(xdft5));
fprintf('Delta:Maximum occurs at %f Hz.\n',freq5(I));
```

A3 PURPOSE OF THIS CODE IS TO DETECT THE STATE OF THE MIND OF A PATIENT USING THE EEG DATA COLLECTED FROM THE PATENT. THIS MATLAB PROGRAM DETECTS THE PATIENT'S STATE OF MIND AND CLASSIFIES IT INTO TWO STATES I.E. EITHER IT IS IN THE STATE OF ANAESTHESIA OR WAKE-UP STATE BY ANALYZING THE FREQUENCY, AMPLITUDE, POWER SPECTRAL DENSITY AVERAGE POWER OF THE COMPONENTS GAMMA, BETA, ALPHA, THETA, AND DELTA WAVES OBTAINED FROM THE EEG OF THE PATENT

```
clear all
close all
clc
%part 1
Fs=128; %sampling frequency as we are using just 128 samplesper second
fileID = fopen('Subject_1.txt','r'); %open Subject_1.txt file in read mode
this_line=0;
var1={}; %initilization of array
while this_line ~=-1%read till end of line of array
this_line=fgetl(fileID); %returns the next line of the specified file, removing the newline characters
if this_line ~=-1%when end of line occure
var1=[var1;this_line]; %concatenate of new line with all the pervious lines and loading into MATLAB array this will result all the text file in into arrays indexes each line make one index
end
end
var2=var1(220); %slect the specfied line whose spectrum you wanted to observe. this will select specfied index of 129*1 array
dlmwrite('myFile.txt',var2,'delimiter','','roffset',1); %this will write the specfied index of array into a text file
fileID = fopen('myFile.txt','r'); %again we open the created file in read mode
commas = char(44); %as our text file is separated by commas so we need the ACII of commas to delete them from text
sizeA = [1 Inf]; %give the size of array
[A] = fscanf(fileID,['%d' commas], sizeA); %make array of decimal data type with specified size and remove commas from text
% %%%filters
%part 3%%power spectrum of delta
fp1=0; %pass band frequecy of delta
fs1=3.75; %stop band frequency of delta
Rs1=.0001; %stop band ripples of delta
Rp1=0.057501127785; %pass band ripples of delta
wn1=[fp1 fs1]/(Fs/2); %retrun the normalize frequency
```

```
[N1, F1, A1, W1] = firpmord(wn1, [0 1], [Rp1,Rs1]); %see the description of fuction
b1 = firpm(N1, F1, A1, W1); %return coefficients of fir filter
Hd1 = dfilt.dffir(b1); %design a filter for the coefficients
x1=filter(Hd1,A); %filter data with the designed filter
L=10;
Q1 = 2^nextpow2(L); %number of fft points
j1 = fft(x1,Q1)/L; %take Fourier transform
Sam1=j1(1:Q1/2); %take Q/2 samples of J
N1=128; %number of samples to find avreage power
PSD1=periodogram(Sam1); %power spectrum density
avg1=sum(PSD1)/N1%average power of delta
f1 = (0:length(PSD1)-1)/(Fs/length(PSD1)); %frequency vector
subplot(221)
plot(f1,PSD1)
title('delta power spectrum')
xlabel('frequacy(Hz)-->')
ylabel('amplitude(db)-->')
%theta
Fs21=3.75;
Fp21=4;
Fp22=7;
Fs22=7.75;
Rs21=.001;
Rs22=.0001;
Rp21=0.057501127785;
wn2=[Fs21 Fp21 Fp22 Fs22]/(Fs/2);
[N2, F2, A2, W2] = firpmord(wn2, [0 1 0], [Rs21, Rp21,Rs22]);
b2 = firpm(N2, F2, A2, W2);
Hd2 = dfilt.dffir(b2);
x2=filter(Hd2,A);
L=10;
Q2 = 2^nextpow2(L);
j2 = fft(x2,Q2)/L;
Sam2=j2(1:Q2/2);
PSD2=periodogram(Sam2); %power spectrum density
avg2=sum(PSD2)/N1%average power of theta
f2 = (0:length(PSD2)-1)/(Fs/length(PSD2));
subplot(222)
plot(f2,PSD2)
title('theta power spectrum')
xlabel('frequacy(Hz)-->')
ylabel('amplitude-->')
%alpha
Fs31=7.75;
```

```
fp31=8;
fp32=13;
fs32=13.5;
Rs31=.001;
Rs32=.0001;
Rp3=0.057501127785;
wn3=[Fs31 fp31 fp32 fs32]/(Fs/2);
[N3, F3, A3, W3] = firpmord(wn3, [0 1 0], [Rs31, Rp3,Rs32]);
b3 = firpm(N3, F3, A3, W3);
Hd3 = dfilt.dffir(b3);
x3=filter(Hd3,A);
L=10;
Q3 = 2^nextpow2(L); % Next power of 2 from length of x3
j3 = fft(x3,Q3)/L;
Sam3=j3(1:Q3/2);
PSD3=periodogram(Sam3); %power spectrum density
avg3=sum(PSD3)/N1%average power of alpha
f3 = (0:length(PSD3)-1)/(Fs/length(PSD3));
subplot(223)
plot(f3,PSD3)
title('Alpha power spectrum')
xlabel('frequacy(Hz)-->')
ylabel('amplitude(db)-->')
% % % %beta
Fs41=13.5;
fp41=14;
fp42=29.5;
fs42=30;
Rs41=.001;
Rs42=.0001;
Rp4=0.057501127785;
wn4=[Fs41 fp41 fp42 fs42]/(Fs/2);
[N4, F4, A4, W4] = firpmord(wn4, [0 1 0], [Rs41, Rp4,Rs42]);
b4 = firpm(N4, F4, A4, W4);
Hd4 = dfilt.dffir(b4);
x4=filter(Hd4,A);
L=10;
Q4= 2^nextpow2(L);
j4 = fft(x4,Q4)/L;
Sam4=j4(1:Q4/2);
PSD4=periodogram(Sam4); %power spectrum density
avg4=sum(PSD4)/N1%average power of beta
f4 = (0:length(PSD4)-1)/(Fs/length(PSD4));
subplot(224)
plot(f4,PSD4)
```

```
title('beta power spectrum')
xlabel('frequacy(Hz)-->')
ylabel('amplitude(db)-->')
if(avg1>41.0777)&&(avg2>.5779)&&(avg3>.2715)&&(avg4>1.8993)
fprintf('patent is awake')
else
fprintf('Patent is Anesthetized\n')
end

clear all
close all
clc
%part 1
fileID = fopen('Subject_1.txt','r');
this_line=0;
var1={};
while this_line ~=-1
this_line=fgetl(fileID);
if this_line ~=-1
var1=[var1;this_line];
end
end
var2=var1(420); %enter row number you want to analyze
dlmwrite('myFile.txt',var2,'delimiter','','roffset',1);
fileID = fopen('myFile.txt','r');
commas = char(44);
sizeA = [1 Inf];
[A] = fscanf(fileID,['%d' commas],sizeA);
fs=500;
A=A';
Z=A(129,1);
if Z==0
fprintf('patient wake\n')
else
fprintf('patient is in Anesthetized\n')
end
%part 2
j=fft(A,1024);
oo=length(j);
L=(0:oo-1)*(fs/oo);
subplot(331)
plot(L,20*log((j)))
title('spectrum of original data')
xlabel('frequacy(Hz)-->')
ylabel('amplitude(db)-->')
```

```
%%%filters
%part 3%%delta
Fp=.5;
Fs=3.75;
Rp=0.057501127785;
wn=[Fp, Fs]/(fs/2);
fs=500;
Rs=0.0001;
[Or,F,po,w] = firpmord(wn, [1 0], [Rp, Rs]);
b1 = firpm(Or, F, po, w);
F1 = dfilt.dffir(b1);
x1=filter(F1,A);
subplot(332)
ts=1;
t=0:ts:128;
plot(t,x1,'r')
title('delta time domain')
xlabel('time(S)-->')
ylabel('amplitude(db)-->')
j=fft(x1,1024);
oo=length(j);
L=(0:oo-1)*(fs/oo);
subplot(333)
plot(L,20*log((j)));
title('delta spectrum')
xlabel('frequacy(Hz)-->')
ylabel('amplitude(db)-->')
%theta
Fs1=3.75;
fp1=4;
fp2=7;
fs2=7.75;
Rs1=.001;
Rs2=.0001;
Rp=0.057501127785;
wn=[Fs1 fp1 fp2 fs2]/(fs/2);
[Or, F, po, w] = firpmord(wn, [0 1 0], [Rs1, Rp,Rs2]);
b1 = firpm(Or, F, po, w);
F1 = dfilt.dffir(b1);
x1=filter(F1,A);
subplot(334)
ts=1;
t=0:ts:128;
plot(t,x1,'r')
title('theta in time domain')
```

```
xlabel('time(S)-->')
ylabel('amplitude(db)-->')
j=fft(x1,1024);
oo=length(j);
L=(0:oo-1)*(fs/oo);
subplot(335)
plot(L,20*log((j)))
title('theta spectrum')
xlabel('frequacy(Hz)-->')
ylabel('amplitude(db)-->')
%alpha
Fs1=7.75;
fp1=8;
fp2=13;
fs2=13.5;
Rs1=.001;
Rs2=.0001;
Rp=0.057501127785;
wn=[Fs1 fp1 fp2 fs2]/(fs/2);
[Or, F, po, w] = firpmord(wn, [0 1 0], [Rs1, Rp,Rs2]);
b1 = firpm(Or, F, po, w);
F1 = dfilt.dffir(b1);
x1=filter(F1,A);
subplot(336)
ts=1;
t=0:ts:128;
plot(t,x1,'r')
title('Alpha in time domain')
xlabel('time(S)-->')
ylabel('amplitude(db)-->')
j=fft(x1,1024);
oo=length(j);
L=(0:oo-1)*(fs/oo);
subplot(337)
plot(L,20*log((j)))
title('Alpha spectrum')
xlabel('frequacy(Hz)-->')
ylabel('amplitude(db)-->')
%beta
Fs1=13.5;
fp1=14;
fp2=29.5;
fs2=30;
Rs1=.001;
Rs2=.0001;
```

```
Rp=0.057501127785;
wn=[Fs1 fp1 fp2 fs2]/(fs/2);
[Or, F, po, w] = firpmord(wn, [0 1 0], [Rs1, Rp,Rs2]);
b1 = firpm(Or, F, po, w);
F1 = dfilt.dffir(b1);
x1=filter(F1,A);
subplot(338)
ts=1;
t=0:ts:128;
plot(t,x1,'r')
title('beta in time domain')
xlabel('time(S)-->')
ylabel('amplitude(db)-->')
j=fft(x1,1024);
oo=length(j);
L=(0:oo-1)*(fs/oo);
subplot(339)
plot(L,20*log((j)))
title('beta spectrum')
xlabel('frequacy(Hz)-->')
ylabel('amplitude(db)-->')

clear all
close all
clc
%part 1
fileID = fopen('Subject_2.txt','r');
this_line=0;
var1={};
while this_line ~=-1
this_line=fgetl(fileID);
if this_line ~=-1
var1=[var1;this_line];
end
end
var2=var1(250); %enter row number you want to analyze
dlmwrite('myFile.txt',var2,'delimiter','','roffset',1);
fileID = fopen('myFile.txt','r');
commas = char(44);
sizeA = [1 Inf];
[A] = fscanf(fileID,['%d' commas],sizeA);
fs=500;
A=A';
Z=A(129,1);
if Z==0
```

```
fprintf('patient wake\n')
else
fprintf('patient is in Anesthetized\n')
end
%part 2
j=fft(A);
oo=length(j);
L=(0:oo-1)*(fs/oo);
subplot(331)
stem(L,20*log((j)))
title('spectrum of original data')
xlabel('frequacy(Hz)-->')
ylabel('amplitude(db)-->')
%%%filters
%part 3%%delta
Fp=.5;
Fs=3.75;
Rp=0.057501127785;
wn=[Fp, Fs]/(fs/2);
fs=500;
Rs=0.0001;
[Or,F,po,w] = firpmord(wn, [1 0], [Rp, Rs]);
b1 = firpm(Or, F, po, w);
F1 = dfilt.dffir(b1);
x1=filter(F1,A);
subplot(332)
ts=1;
t=0:ts:128;
stem(t,x1,'r')
title('delta time domain')
xlabel('time(S)-->')
ylabel('amplitude(db)-->')
j=fft(x1);
oo=length(j);
L=(0:oo-1)*(fs/oo);
subplot(333)
stem(L,20*log((j)));
title('delta spectrum')
xlabel('frequacy(Hz)-->')
ylabel('amplitude(db)-->')
%theta
Fs1=3.75;
fp1=4;
fp2=7;
fs2=7.75;
```

```
Rs1=.001;
Rs2=.0001;
Rp=0.057501127785;
wn=[Fs1 fp1 fp2 fs2]/(fs/2);
[Or, F, po, w] = firpmord(wn, [0 1 0], [Rs1, Rp,Rs2]);
b1 = firpm(Or, F, po, w);
F1 = dfilt.dffir(b1);
x1=filter(F1,A);
subplot(334)
ts=1;
t=0:ts:128;
stem(t,x1,'r')
title('theta in time domain')
xlabel('time(S)-->')
ylabel('amplitude(db)-->')
j=fft(x1);
oo=length(j);
L=(0:oo-1)*(fs/oo);
subplot(335)
stem(L,20*log((j)))
title('theta spectrum')
xlabel('frequacy(Hz)-->')
ylabel('amplitude(db)-->')
%alpha
Fs1=7.75;
fp1=8;
fp2=13;
fs2=13.5;
Rs1=.001;
Rs2=.0001;
Rp=0.057501127785;
wn=[Fs1 fp1 fp2 fs2]/(fs/2);
[Or, F, po, w] = firpmord(wn, [0 1 0], [Rs1, Rp,Rs2]);
b1 = firpm(Or, F, po, w);
F1 = dfilt.dffir(b1);
x1=filter(F1,A);
subplot(336)
ts=1;
t=0:ts:128;
stem(t,x1,'r')
title('Alpha in time domain')
xlabel('time(S)-->')
ylabel('amplitude(db)-->')
```

```
j=fft(x1);
oo=length(j);
L=(0:oo-1)*(fs/oo);
subplot(337)
stem(L,20*log((j)))
title('Alpha spectrum')
xlabel('frequacy(Hz)-->')
ylabel('amplitude(db)-->')
%beta
Fs1=13.5;
fp1=14;
fp2=29.5;
fs2=30;
Rs1=.001;
Rs2=.0001;
Rp=0.057501127785;
wn=[Fs1 fp1 fp2 fs2]/(fs/2);
[Or, F, po, w] = firpmord(wn, [0 1 0], [Rs1, Rp,Rs2]);
b1 = firpm(Or, F, po, w);
F1 = dfilt.dffir(b1);
x1=filter(F1,A);
subplot(338)
ts=1;
t=0:ts:128;
stem(t,x1,'r')
title('beta in time domain')
xlabel('time(S)-->')
ylabel('amplitude(db)-->')
j=fft(x1);
oo=length(j);
L=(0:oo-1)*(fs/oo);
subplot(339)
stem(L,20*log((j)))
title('beta spectrum')
xlabel('frequacy(Hz)-->')
ylabel('amplitude(db)-->')
```

A4 MATLAB CODE FOR DETECTION OF BLINKS FROM EEG DATA

A4.1 Main Function

```
%{
==========================================================
Title:A Method to Detect Blink from the EEG Signal
Author: Narayan Panigrahi, Center for AI and Robotics(CAIR), Bangalore,
India, email: npanigrahi7@gmail.com
```

Amarnath De, student, Jadavpur University, amarnathde1992work@gmail.com
Somnath Roy, student, Jadavpur University, somroymail@gmail.com

```
=================================================================
%}
%%
%EEG Signal aquired using EEGLAB Toolbox v14.1.2b
%A1 channel No 31 is taken for blink detection
channel1 = sangeeta(31,:);
t = 1:size(channel1,2);
%Moving average taken with Lead = 10, Lag = 20, alpha = 1%
This is done to remove the local variations in the signal
[modified_long,modified_short] = movavg(channel1,10,20,1);
%%
%Takeing the differential of the signal to obtain the gradient
steps = 1;
grad = zeros(int32(size(modified_short,2)/steps));
fori = 1:(size(modified_short,1))/steps-1
   grad(i) = (modified_short(i+steps) - modified_short(i))/steps;
end
%%
%Calculating the parameters of the Modified threshold function
mod_val = abs(grad);
max_mod = max(mod_val);
c = 0.3;
thresh = max_mod*c;
%apply moving averge using the same parameters
[ None,smooth_grad] = movavg(grad,10,20,1);
%calling the Threshold function
[squared,blinks,count_blinks] = thresh_sign(transpose(smooth_grad),...
           -thresh,thresh);
%Function to highlight the blinks in the original signal
plot_blinks(blinks,count_blinks, channel1)
%%
%plot the result
subplot(4,1,1)
grid on
plot(modified_short, 'LineWidth',1.5)
title('Signal after applying moving average of Lead = 10 Lag = 20Alpha= 1')
xlabel('Time')
ylabel('Amplitude(uV)')
subplot(4,1,2)
plot(grad,'LineWidth',1.5)
title('Gradient change of the above signal using 1st order derivative')
xlabel('Time')
```

```
ylabel('Gradient')
subplot(4,1,3)
plot(squared,'LineWidth',1.5)
title('Result After Thresholding ')
xlabel('Time')
ylabel('Amplitude')
```

A4.2 Threshold Function

```
%{===========================================================
Title:A Method to Detect Blink from the EEG Signal
Author: Narayan Panigrahi, Center for AI and Robotics(CAIR), Bangalore,
India, email: npanigrahi7@gmail.com
Amarnath De, student, Jadavpur University, amarnathde1992work@gmail.com
Somnath Roy, student, Jadavpur University, somroymail@gmail.com
===========================================================%}
function [ y, blinks,count_blinks] = thresh_sign( x, lower_thresh,...
high_thresh)
%thresh_sign: This function determines the blinks.
%This function determines the blink if the the gradient crosses the higher
%and lower threshold in quick successions otherwise it won't.
%Input:gradient signal, lower threshold and higher threshold
%Output: squared signal, array containing the start and end of blinks
%and number of blinks
y = zeros(size(x));
plot(x)
pause
start=0;
ending=0;
flag = 0;
blinks = zeros(2,1);
count_blinks = 1;
fori = 2:size(x,2)
if( x(i)>high_thresh)

   y(i) = 2*high_thresh;
if(x(i-1)<=high_thresh&& x(i-1)>0)
if(flag == 1) % not a blink so set flag to 0
      flag = 0;
elseif(flag==0)
      start = i-1; %record the time of blink start
      flag = 1; %set flag to signify the start of blink
end
end
```

```
elseif(x(i)<=high_thresh&& x(i)>0)
   y(i) = high_thresh;
elseif(x(i)<0 && x(i)>lower_thresh)
   y(i) = lower_thresh;
if(x(i-1)<=lower_thresh)
if(flag == 1)
       ending = i-1; %record the time of blink ends
       flag = 0; %set flag to signify the end of blink
       blinks(:,count_blinks) = [start;ending];
count_blinks = count_blinks+1;
end
end
elseif(x(i)<=lower_thresh)
       y(i) = 2*lower_thresh;
end
end
end
```

A4.3 Plot Blink Function

```
%{==========================================================
Title:A Method to Detect Blink from the EEG Signal
Author: Narayan Panigrahi, Center for AI and Robotics(CAIR), Bangalore,
India, email: npanigrahi7@gmail.com
Amarnath De, student, Jadavpur University, amarnathde1992work@gmail.com
Somnath Roy, student, Jadavpur University, somroymail@gmail.com
==========================================================%}
function [] = plot_blinks( blinks, count_blinks, channel1)
%plot_blinks: Highlights the blinks in the original signal
count = 1;
start = blinks(1,1);
ending = blinks(2,1);
subplot(4,1,4)
for t = 2:size(channel1,2)
if(t>=start && t <= ending)
   plot(t-1:t,channel1(t-1:t),'r','LineWidth',1.5)
   hold on
else
   plot(t-1:t,channel1(t-1:t),'LineWidth',1.5)
   hold on
end
if (t>ending && count<count_blinks-1)%if plot completes one blink
     count = count +1;
     start = blinks(1,count);
     ending = blinks(2,count);
```

```
end

end
title('Original Signals with Highlighted Blinks')
xlabel('Time')
ylabel('Amplitude(uV)')
```

A5 MATLAB CODE FOR DETECTION OF SACCADE AND FIX

A5.1 Main Function

```
X1=115712;
X2=116712;
%=========================Wavelet Decomposition============

A1_raw=double(A(32,X1:X2)); % Selecting EOG1 channel from raw data.
t=(1:(X2-X1)+1);
A1=wavdecomp( A1_raw); % Wavelet Decomposition to remove baseline.
%A1 = A1_raw; % Level=12 IDFT upto level 8.
subplot(211)
plot(t,A1_raw,'LineWidth',1.5)
xlabel('Time[ms]')
ylabel('Original Signal Amplitude')
grid on
title('Raw EEG Signal','FontSize',16)
subplot(212)
plot(t,A1,'LineWidth',1.5)
xlabel('Time[ms]')
ylabel('Amplitude')
grid on
title('Baseline Removed Signal','FontSize',16) %Comparison Plot of baseline
%removed signal.

%================Median Filter and Wavelet Denoising===========

A1_medfilt=medfilt1(A1,19,74); % Applying Median filter of 19th order with
% window of 74ms.

[A1_wden] = wden(A1,'sqtwolog','s','one',1,'sym1'); % Applying symlet
%wavelet denoising to remove noise
A1_final=(A1_medfilt+A1_wden)/2; % Averaging both to get final signal.

figure,plot(t,A1,t,A1_medfilt,t,A1_wden,t,A1_final,'LineWidth',1.5)
xlabel('Time[ms]')
ylabel('Amplitude')
```

```
title('Baseline Removed Signal vs Median Filter Applied Signal Vs Wavelet
Denoised Signal vs Resultant Signal','FontSize',16)
legend('Baseline Removed Signal','Median Filter Applied Signal',...
'Wavelet Denoised Signal','Resultant Signal', 'FontSize',18)

figure,plot(t,A1,t,A1_final,'LineWidth',2)
title('A1 vs A1_final','FontSize',14)
xlabel('Time[ms]')
ylabel('Amplitude')
legend('Baseline Removed Signal',' Median Filter Applied Signal')

%============================Continuous Wavelet Transform=====
subplot(211)
A1_cwt=cwt(A1_final,20,'haar'); % Continuous 'Haar' Wavelet Transform to
% find abrupt change in voltage
% (saccades and blinks)
plot(A1_cwt,'LineWidth',2)
title('Cwt Coefficients','FontSize',16)
xlabel('Time[ms]')
ylabel('Coefficients Amplitude')

subplot(212)
plot(t,A1_final,'LineWidth',2)
title('Resulting Signal','FontSize',16)
xlabel('Time[ms]')
ylabel('Amplitude')

%======================saccad Detection=====================

threshold = 25;
[start_pos,ending_pos, start_neg, ending_neg] = plot_thresh(A1_cwt,...
  A1_final,threshold); %Applying threshold on A_cwt to find abrupt changes in
%the signal
pos_points = [start_pos; ending_pos];
neg_points = [start_neg; ending_neg];
%max peaks
pos = find_max(pos_points, A1_cwt); % Detecting the +ve peak coefficients
neg = find_max(neg_points, -A1_cwt);% Detecting the -ve peak coefficients

figure,subplot(211)
plot(t,A1_cwt,pos,A1_cwt(pos),'*g',neg,A1_cwt(neg),'*r',...
  t,threshold,'--m',t,-threshold,':k','LineWidth',2)
xlabel('Time[ms]')
ylabel('Coefficient Amplitude')
title(...
```

```
'Positive and Negetive Peaks of CWT Coefficients After Thresholding',...
'FontSize',16)
%legend('CWT Coefficients', 'Positive Peaks','Negative Peaks',...
% 'Upper Threshold','Lower Threshold')

subplot(212)
plot(t,A1_raw,pos,A1_raw(pos),'*g',neg,A1_raw(neg),'*r','LineWidth',2)
xlabel('Time[ms]')
ylabel('Original Signal Amplitude')
title('Detected Saccads','FontSize',16)
```

A6 WAVELET DECOMPOSITION FOR REMOVAL OF BASELINE DRIFT IN EEG SIGNALS

```
function [baseline_remove] = wavdecomp( signal)
%Wavelet decomposition for baseline drift removal
wave = 'rbio6.8';
t1 = 1:size(signal,2);
level = 12;
[c0,i0] = wavedec(signal,level,wave);
cD1 = detcoef(c0,i0,1);
cD2 = detcoef(c0,i0,2);
cD3 = detcoef(c0,i0,3);
cD4 = detcoef(c0,i0,4);
cD5 = detcoef(c0,i0,5);
cA5 =appcoef(c0,i0,wave,5);
D1 = wrcoef('d',c0,i0,wave,1);
D2 = wrcoef('d',c0,i0,wave,2);
D3 = wrcoef('d',c0,i0,wave,3);
D4 = wrcoef('d',c0,i0,wave,4);
D5 = wrcoef('d',c0,i0,wave,5);
D6 = wrcoef('d',c0,i0,wave,6);
D7 = wrcoef('d',c0,i0,wave,7);
D8 = wrcoef('d',c0,i0,wave,8);
D9 = wrcoef('d',c0,i0,wave,9);
D10 = wrcoef('d',c0,i0,wave,10);
D11 = wrcoef('d',c0,i0,wave,11);
D12 = wrcoef('d',c0,i0,wave,12);
A12 = wrcoef('a',c0,i0,wave,12);

baseline_remove = D1+D2+D3+D4+D5+D6+D7+D8+D9;

figure,plot(t1,signal,t1,baseline_remove,'LineWidth',1)
xlabel('Time[ms]')
ylabel('Amplitude')
```

```
title('Flitered Data After Baseline Removal','FontSize',14)
legend('Original','Baseline Removed')

end
```

A6.1 Plotting the Threshold on a CWT Transformed Function

```
function [start_pos ,ending_pos, start_neg, ending_neg ] = plot_thresh( X_cwt,
X_final ,thresh )
%Ploting The threshold on CWT transformed Function
start_pos=[];
ending_pos =[];
start_neg=[];
ending_neg =[];
size(X_cwt,2);
flag_p = 0;
flag_n = 0;
for j = 2 : size(X_cwt,2)-1

if(X_cwt(j)>=thresh)

if(X_cwt(j-1)<thresh)

    start_pos =cat(2,start_pos, j);
    s_prev_p = j;
    flag_p =1;

end

if(X_cwt(j+1)<thresh)

if(flag_p == 1 && ((j-s_prev_p)>1) )
   ending_pos = cat(2,ending_pos,j);
   flag_p = 0;
else
    start_pos = start_pos(1:size(start_pos,2)-1);
end
end
end
if(X_cwt(j)<=-thresh)

if(X_cwt(j-1)>-thresh)

    start_neg =cat(2,start_neg, j);
    s_prev_n = j;
```

```
    flag_n =1;
end
if(X_cwt(j+1)>-thresh)

if(flag_n == 1 && ((j-s_prev_n)>1) )
    ending_neg = cat(2,ending_neg,j);
    flag_n = 0;

else
         start_neg = start_neg(1:size(start_neg,2)-1);
               end
          end
     end
end

t = 1:size(X_final,2);

figure,plot(t,X_cwt,'LineWidth',2) ; hold on
plot(start_pos,X_cwt(start_pos),'r*') ; hold on
plot(ending_pos,X_cwt(ending_pos),'g*') ; hold on
plot(ending_neg,X_cwt(ending_neg),'b*') ; hold on
plot(start_neg,X_cwt(start_neg),'y*') ; hold on
plot(t,thresh,'--m',t,-thresh,'--k'); title('Thresholding on CWT Coefficients
','FontSize',14)
end
```

A6.2 Finding the Positive and Negative Peaks of a CWT Transformed Signal

```
function [ peak_indices ] = find_max( points, x_cwt)
%Finding the positive and Negative peaks of CWT transformed Signal
peak_indices = zeros(1,size(points,2));
for i=1:size(points,2)
   start = points(1,i);
   ending = points(2,i);
if(ending-start>1)
   [C,I] = max(x_cwt(start:ending));
   peak_indices(1,i) = start+I;
        end
end
%t = 1:size(x_cwt,2);
%figure,plot(t,x_cwt,peak_indices,x_cwt(peak_indices),'*r')
end
```

Index

Note: **Bold** page numbers refer to tables and *Italic* page numbers refer to figures.

Made in the USA
Las Vegas, NV
19 September 2026

89de79de-092e-419b-b6cb-6f6fa03f8969R01